Visual and Related Disorders in Children

Visual and Related Disorders in Children

Yogesh Shukla

Visiting Professor
National Institute of Medical Sciences, Jaipur

Former Professor
SMS Medical College, Jaipur

CBS Publishers & Distributors Pvt Ltd

New Delhi • Bengaluru • Chennai • Kochi • Kolkata • Mumbai
Bhopal • Bhubaneswar • Hyderabad • Jharkhand • Nagpur • Patna • Pune • Uttarakhand • Dhaka (Bangladesh)

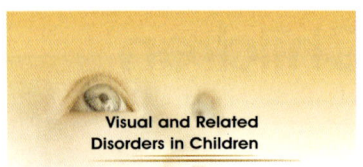

Visual and Related Disorders in Children

ISBN: 978-93-86827-90-6

First Edition: 2020

Published by Satish Kumar Jain and produced by Varun Jain for

CBS Publishers & Distributors Pvt Ltd

4819/XI Prahlad Street, 24 Ansari Road, Daryaganj, New Delhi 110 002, India.
Ph: 23289259, 23266861, 23266867 Website: www.cbspd.com
Fax: 011-23243014 e-mail: delhi@cbspd.com; cbspubs@airtelmail.in.

Corporate Office: 204 FIE, Industrial Area, Patparganj, Delhi 110 092
Ph: 4934 4934 Fax: 4934 4935 e-mail: publishing@cbspd.com; publicity@cbspd.com

Branches

- **Bengaluru:** Seema House 2975, 17th Cross, K.R. Road, Banasankari 2nd Stage, Bengaluru 560 070, Karnataka
  Ph: +91-80-26771678/79 Fax: +91-80-26771680 e-mail: bangalore@cbspd.com
- **Chennai:** 7, Subbaraya Street, Shenoy Nagar, Chennai 600 030, Tamil Nadu
  Ph: +91-44-26680620/26681266 Fax: +91-44-42032115 e-mail: chennai@cbspd.com
- **Kochi:** 42/1325, 1326, Power House Road, Opp KSEB, Power House, Ernakulam 682 018, Kochi, Kerala
  Ph: +91-484-4059061-65 Fax: +91-484-4059065 e-mail: kochi@cbspd.com
- **Kolkata:** 6/B, Ground Floor, Rameswar Shaw Road, Kolkata-700 014, West Bengal
  Ph: +91-33-22891126, 22891127, 22891128 e-mail: kolkata@cbspd.com
- **Mumbai:** 83-C, Dr E Moses Road, Worli, Mumbai-400018, Maharashtra
  Ph: +91-22-24902340/41 Fax: +91-22-24902342 e-mail: mumbai@cbspd.com

Representatives

• **Bhopal**	0-8319310552	• **Bhubaneswar**	0-9911037372	• **Hyderabad**	0-9885175004
• **Jharkhand**	0-9811541605	• **Nagpur**	0-9421945513	• **Patna**	0-9334159340
• **Pune**	0-9623451994	• **Uttarakhand**	0-9716462459	• **Dhaka (Bangladesh)**	01912-003485

Printed at : HT Media Ltd., Greater Noida, UP, India

to
my parents,
who brought me in this world and
made me capable of writing this book

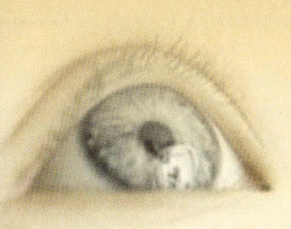

Preface

Going by recent figures, almost 40 million people are blind worldwide. Of which, India has the largest share of 15 million blind persons. Shockingly, 26% of these blind people in India are children, almost 3 million! Strikingly, 80% of the blindness in children is either preventable or treatable.

Almost 20 million children worldwide are suffering from serious vision problems, mostly uncorrected high refractive errors and amblyopia.

The extent to which poor vision hurts children-psychologically, socially, educationally, and economically- is unprecedented and is often underappreciated and overlooked.

The aim of this book is to bring together all the disorders that affect vision in children, directly or indirectly. The initial chapters are dedicated to basic science of vision, with the intention that an ophthalmologist must also be aware of how the vision and neuro-visual system in a child develops, because without a thorough knowledge of visual milestones, assessment of vision and other visual faculties, can be faulty.

Psychological development of a child has been duly stressed in recent times, because visual assessment in a small child depends, upon a large part, on its psychological and cognitive development. Thus, most tests for vision in a small child, take into account the mental age of the child.

One of the most important defect or disorder that affects a child is amblyopia. It is the most common cause of unilateral blindness, and frequently goes unnoticed, owing to it being unilateral in most cases. Path breaking discoveries in the concept of amblyopia, has made a sea change in the overall management and in recovery of vision far beyond the conventional age limit.

Refractive errors, particularly myopia, is a major public health problem all over the world, and in years to come, it will assume an epidemic status. With modest projections, by 2050, half of the world's population will be myopic and one person in every ten, will be at risk of permanent blindness! The chapter on refractive errors, therefore, will open new paradigms for management, especially of myopia.

Certain conditions such as accommodative anomalies and hyper acuity deficiencies, have never been part of clinical ophthalmic examination in child. The reader will be surprised to know that a myriad of ocular complaints stem from disorders which we have never thought of.

Later part of the book is laced with chapters which will highlight so many para-visual conditions which mimic actual vision disorders and are a nightmare as far as management is concerned. Every ophthalmologist must be aware and conversant with these disorders, as they are also in the domain of visual deficiencies.

Lastly, when all is lost, we must endeavour to salvage whatever is remaining. Therefore, an ophthalmologist must also be concerned for a child who has fatefully become blind and be responsible for its rehabilitation.

The book has emerged from long hours of arduous, painstaking, and sincere clinical research and an essence of endurance of plight and pain of children who have needlessly become blind.

Yogesh Shukla

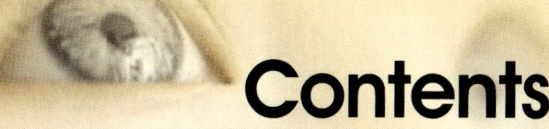

Contents

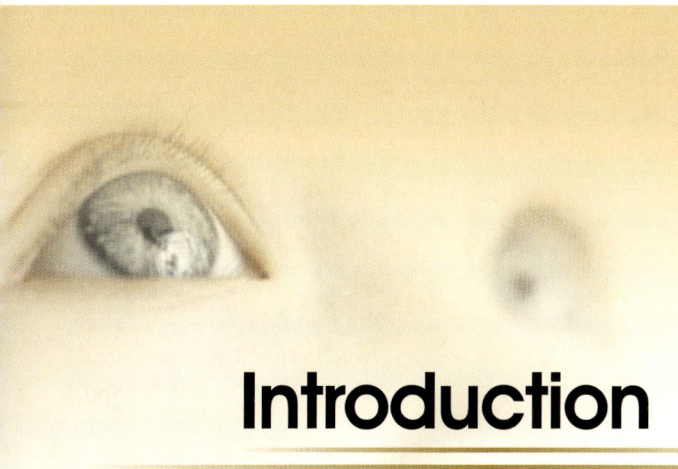

Introduction

Vision science can be defined as the study of vision, the visual system, and the relationship between the two. When we study vision, we use psychophysical and perceptual techniques to describe what we see and how well we see; how good are our spatial and temporal resolutions.

When we journey through the visual system, we come across two different systems complimenting each other. First, the eye where the image is formed and the way it is carried to the visual cortex; and the second, the perceptual capabilities in cortex where we understand and comprehend what we are seeing!

The intent of writing this book is to understand the development of vision, its discrepancies and to demonstrate the methods to solve these defects. But as time and research went into writing the contents, a second thought crept into mind, and that is, the 'perceptual' deficiencies of vision.

Vision, as we know it, comprises of not only the visual acuity or sharpness of vision, but also stereoacuity, contrast sensitivity, color sensations, visual fields, the vision of motion, form recognition, hyperacuity, and so on! Beyond these visual functions, there is another horizon where cognitive perceptions related to vision come into play. Therefore, this book is laced with chapters which will also look into some defects which are indirectly related to vision. It is difficult and may be controversial to relate these discrepancies with vision per se;

but children with these problems come to the ophthalmologist first and understandably it becomes obligatory on our part to understand these defects, to manage them ourselves or in association with other experts.

Since we now know that visual performances of far greater importance than visual acuity exist, which are the finer qualities of vision and help in assessing the gravity of many childhood diseases. It would be prudent, therefore, to describe these visual assets also.

In some chapters, a brief introduction has been given as a tribute to scholars and scientists who have contributed immensely to the knowledge we have acquired and to whom we owe so much!

The development of vision and the visual system from infancy to adulthood is like blossoming of a flower; but ironically we do not get interested in understanding the intricacies of this system. Most of us know that the visual system including the visual cortex develops until teen age only; but in factuality, in some cases, maturation continues well into adulthood. Our attempts should, therefore, continue to explore new horizons of treatment and rationalize the management on individual basis.

We know that 60% of brain is involved with vision, directly or indirectly; and 80% of learning is through sight in the formative years of a child. Therefore, a proper and uneventful visual development is mandatory in early years of life.

A lot of time, energy and research has gone into writing of this book and a sincere attempt has been made by the author for the learner and the learned, to understand vision, the visual system and the many disorders associated with it.

Anatomical Development of the Eye

EMBRYOLOGY

After fertilization of the ovum, cellular mitosis results in the formation of a ball of 12–15 cells, called the *morula*. A fluid-filled cavity now forms within the morula, termed as *blastocyst*, which embeds itself in the uterine mucosa around 6th day of fertilization. The cells continue to divide and accumulate at one pole. The cells of this 'primitive embryoblast' differentiate into two layers—the 'epiblast' and the 'hypoblast'. These two cellular layers bridge the central cavity, thus dividing the blastocyst into the amniotic sac and the yolk sac.

Division and differentiation continues and the epiblast cells give rise to all three definitive germ layers, viz. 'ectoderm', 'mesoderm' and 'endoderm'. The central ectoderm differentiates to form a columnar 'neural ectoderm'. This forms the neural plate, which later develops into the head and brain.

At about 21 days of gestation, previously formed neural folds from neural groove fuse to form the 'neural tube' in the middle of the embryo. At this time, the first signs of developing eye is seen, called the 'optic pit'. The optic pits are seen as invaginations of neural ectoderm on the inner surface of the anterior neural folds.

As the neural folds elevate and approach each other, a specialized population of mesenchyme cells, the 'neural crest' cells develop. Neural crest cells play an important role in eye development because they are the precursors to major eye structures including the corneal stroma, ciliary muscles, iris stroma, choroid, sclera, orbital cartilage and bone.

During the development and closure of the neural groove, the mesoderm develops to form 'somites'. These somites give rise to myoblasts which subsequently form the vasculature in and around the eyes.

Unlike trunk and extremities, orbital cartilage, bone and ocular connective tissue are derived from neural crest tissue, not mesoderm. It is important to remember that 'mesenchyme' is a broad term for any embryonic connective tissue, whereas 'mesoderm' specifically relates to embryonic germ layer. Recent embryologic studies have shown that mesoderm plays a relatively small role in the development of face and eyes. With respect to the eyes, most of the mesenchyme tissues come from the neural crest cells. By end of 3 weeks, neural folds progress to form brain vesicles and then segmentation occurs to form specific parts of the brain, i.e. forebrain, midbrain and hindbrain. It is from the forebrain that bilateral 'evaginations' develop to present as 'optic sulci'. Invagination of the optic sulci creates 'optic vesicles'. The transformation of optic sulci into vesicle is considered to occur concurrently with the closure of anterior neural tube, which is completed by 25th day of gestation (3 mm embryo size).

The neural crest cells populate around this vesicle and ultimately give rise to nearly all the connective tissue of the human eyes. The timing and generation of the optic vesicle has a significant role in the induction and size determination of the palpebral aperture and orbital structures.

At around 26 days of gestation, the surface ectoderm that is in contact with the optic vesicle, thickens to form the 'lens placade'. The lens placade then invaginates with the underlying neural ectoderm. The invaginating neural ectoderm folds onto itself, creating a double layer of neural ectoderm, forming the 'optic cup'. The optic cup eventually differentiates into the 'neurosensory retina' (the inner layer) and the 'pigment epithelium layer' (the outer layer).

Invagination of the optic cup occurs in an eccentric manner progressing from inferior to superior, with ultimate formation of a seam, the 'optic fissure' or 'choroidal fissure'. Mesenchyme of neural crest origin surrounds and fills the optic fissure. At 5 weeks of gestation, the hyloid artery develops from the mesenchyme in the optic fissure and courses from the optic stalk to the lens placade anteriorly. The lens placade now separates from the surface ectoderm before the optic fissure closes.

INTRAOCULAR DEVELOPMENT

The closure of the optic fissure, at the end of 7th week, is an important milestone in the development of the eye. Abnormal or delayed closure of the optic fissure results in an inferior coloboma often with microphthalmic eyes. At this stage of 7–8 weeks, the neurosensory retina and pigment epithelium are in approximation, the optic nerve is developing, and the lens vesicle is separating from the cornea to form the anterior chamber. The mesenchyme of neural origin around the primitive retina develops into choroid and the sclera. Around this developing globe, myoblasts of mesodermal origin arrange in linear fashion and are precursors of future extraocular muscles. The eyelids emerge as small buds above and below the globe. As the lens placade invaginates, it forms a hollow center and becomes the 'lens vesicle'. Detachment of the lens placade, now lens vesicle, occurs around 5th week and is the hallmark of formation of chambers within the eye. Failure of proper separation of lens vesicle from the surface ectoderm is one of the characteristics of a teratogenic–induced 'dysgenesis' of the anterior segment of the eye.

Applied anatomy: Anterior lenticonus, anterior capsular cataract, and anterior chamber cleavage syndromes are the result of faulty keratolenticular separation.

Following separation, the lens vesicle gets surrounded by a layer of basal lamina, the lens capsule. At approximately 38–40 days of gestation (6 weeks), the cells of posterior lens vesicle lengthen to fill the vesicle, loose their nuclei and most of their intracellular organelles. It has been found that amazingly retinal anlage promotes primary lens fibre formation. The retina develops independently while the lens appears to rely on the retina for cytodifferentiation. The primitive lens, filled with the primary lens fibres, is the 'embryonic lens nucleus'. In adult, the primary embryonic nucleus is the central round, slightly dark sphere within the 'Y' sutures. Anterior lens epithelial cells remain cuboidal and are mitotic throughout life, giving rise to future fetal and adult lens fibres. The anterior lens cells gradually migrate to the lens periphery (the equator), and they elongate to form secondary lens fibres. These secondary lens fibres course anteriorly and posteriorly around the embryonic nucleus to meet at the centre of lens, the poles. These early lens fibres have blunt ends, so when they meet they form a loose adherence and produce the 'Y' sutures. At birth, the lens is entirely made of nucleus and minimal cortex. The cortex, then, continues to form from the anterior lens fibres throughout life, albeit at a very slow pace.

After separation of the lens vesicle, the overlying surface ectoderm forms the corneal epithelium and then secretes a thick matrix, producing the 'corneal stroma'. Neural crest cells then migrate between lens vesicle and corneal epithelium, filling the anterior chamber and forming the 'corneal endothelium'. The iris develops from the cells of anterior optic cup, iris stroma from the mesenchymal neural crest cells and the two layers of epithelium from the neural ectoderm. The smooth muscles of the iris develop from differentiation of neural ectoderm. The pupillary constrictor and the dilator are only muscles in the body of ectodermal origin.

Differentiation and separation continues in the cells present in the anterior chamber until a cavity, primitive anterior chamber forms. Discrepancies in the separation of this tissue are the harbinger of number of disorders belonging to the 'anterior chamber dysgenesis' syndromes.

The choroid and the sclera are derived from the mesenchymal tissue of neural crest origin. By approximately 12 weeks of gestation, the choroid and sclera have enveloped the optic stalk. The lamina cribrosa consists of cells that have penetrated the optic nerve. By 16 weeks of gestation, the vasculature of the choroid begins to take shape with the choriocapillaries forming, anastomosing with the short posterior ciliary arteries and ultimately joining in the four vortex veins.

DEVELOPMENT OF THE RETINA

Our primary focus, as regards vision, is the development of the retina and the optic nerve. As already mentioned, the retina develops from the neural ectoderm with the outer pigment epithelium (RPE) developing from the outer layer and the neurosensory retina developing from the inner layer of the optic cup. Bruch's membrane, the basal lamina of the pigment epithelium, begins to emerge by 4th week and is well developed by 6th week of gestation.

By 4 months (16 weeks) of gestation, the RPE cells take on their hexagonal shape and develop 'microvilli', which interdigitate with projections from the photoreceptor cells of the inner retina.

By about 8th week, proliferation of cells of inner neuro-sensory retina commences with formation of inner and outer neuroblastic layers, and consequently differentiation of the ganglion cells giving rise to primitive nerve fibre layer.

At about 6 weeks of gestation, axons from the developing ganglion cells pass through the vacuolated spaces of the inner wall of the optic stalk. Simultaneously, 'hyloid artery' develops in the centre of the primitive optic nerve. A glial sheath forms around the hyloid artery and along with the regression of hyaloid arteries the glial tissue also regresses. 'Bergmeister's papilla represents the remnants of this glial tissue. These glial cells migrate to the optic stalk, accumulate there and form the primitive 'optic disc'. These glial cells which form the glial part of the lamina cribrosa, come from the optic stalk which is of neural ectodermal in origin. Later, mesenchymal portion of the disc develops from the neural 'crest' cells.

By 3rd month of gestation, the optic nerve shifts nasally as temporal aspect of the globe enlarges.

Myelination of the optic nerve starts at the chiasma at about 7 months of gestation and progresses towards the eye. Normally, myelination stops at the optic disc, one month post natal. Myelination of retinal nerve fibres occur, if the process of myelination continues past the optic disc. Reason for 'retinal myelination' is explained as an 'ectopic' phenomenon and is associated with high myopia and amblyopia (Figs 1.1 to 1.3).

RETINAL VASCULATURE

It is important to understand the time bound development of retinal vasculature as this has bearing on the prematurity of birth. The central retinal artery grows from the optic disc to

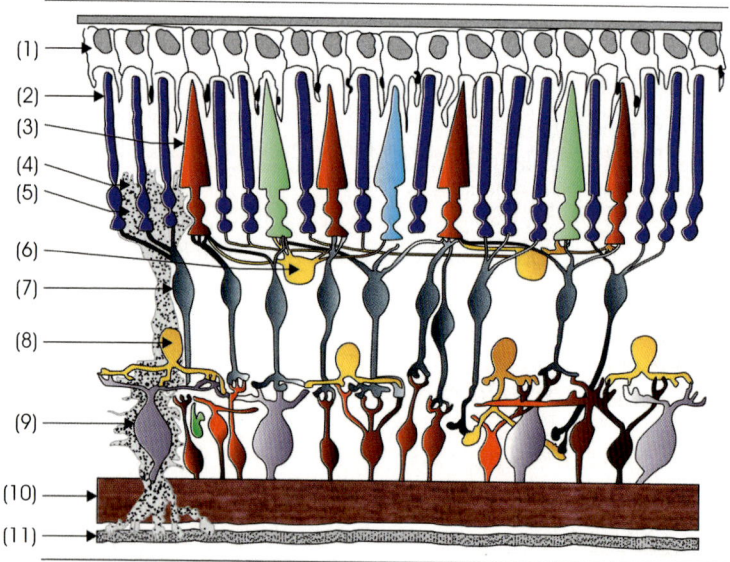

(1) Pigment epithelium; (2) Rods; (3) Cones; (4) Outer limiting membrane; (5) Müller cells; (6) Horizontal cells; (7) Bipolar cells; (8) Amacrine cells; (9) Ganglion cells; (10) Nerve fiber layer; (11) Inner limiting membrane.

Fig. 1.1: Depiction of retinal layers.

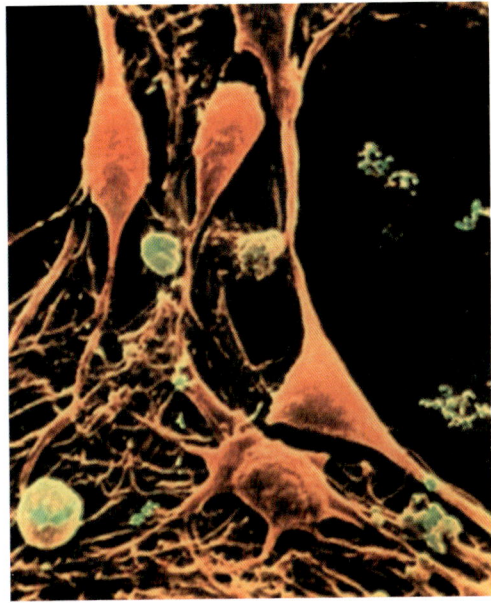

Fig. 1.2: Photomicrograph of amacrine cells of retina

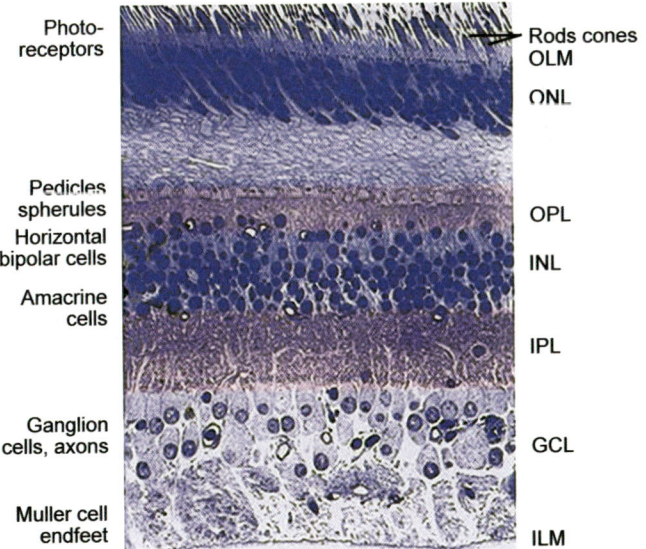

Photo-receptors	Rods cones
	OLM
	ONL
Pedicles spherules	OPL
Horizontal bipolar cells	INL
Amacrine cells	IPL
Ganglion cells, axons	GCL
Muller cell endfeet	ILM

Fig. 1.3: Light micrograph of a vertical section through central human retina

the retinal periphery forming the nasal and temporal arcades. Between 5 and 6 months of gestation, the retinal arcades have progressed to the equator of the eye. By this time, the long and short posterior ciliary arteries have developed with the long ciliary supplying the anterior segment while the short ciliary supplying the choroid. The retinal vessels grow faster towards the nasal retina; even at full term birth, there is a small crescent of temporal retina devoid of vessels. The fact that a newborn infant has an immature temporal retina, may explain scattered cases of ROP even in a full term birth.

Applied anatomy: Oxygen affects 'angiogenesis' and seems to play a role in stimulating or retarding vascular growth. Vascular endothelial growth is promoted by low oxygen tension and is inhibited by high oxygen tension. These findings give rise to the hypothesis that 'retinopathy of prematurity' is secondary to an increased oxygen concentration which results in inhibition or 'retraction' of the peripheral capillary vasculature. This retraction of the vessels results in retinal 'hypoxia' and consequent secondary endothelial cell growth and 'neovascularization'.

By 6 months of gestation, all structures in and around the eye have formed including lids and orbital adnexa. The lid fissure begins to take shape with the separation of the lids. From now on, development and maturation of the structures of the eye continue till birth.

POSTNATAL DEVELOPMENT OF RETINA

Since vision is directly related to the development of retina and visual pathways, it would be relevant to follow the development of these structures in the immediate postnatal life. Of all the structures of the eye, the 'macula' is the least developed at birth. The peripheral retina is comparatively well developed histologically and functionally at birth.

After birth, the macula dramatically develops by 4 years of life, wherein the vision assumes its normal level of functioning. Most notable changes are in macular pigmentation, annular ring development, foveal reflex and cone photoreceptor maturation.

Ophthalmoscopic studies of premature birth infants showed that macular pigmentation is not evident before 33 weeks of gestation. Between 34 and 35 weeks, pigmentation appears in the pigment epithelial cells, producing a dark red appearance, that is quite distinct from the surrounding retina. The pigment epithelial cells at macula become narrower, taller, and more tightly packed and are accountable for the dark appearance. The yellow xanthophyllic pigment usually found in adult retina is not present in neonates. This pigment originates from the 'dietary carotenoids' and appears later in life and gradually increases with age. The parafoveal capillary-free zone also contributes to the typical appearance of macula.

The 'annular ring' at macula, a prominent ophthalmoscopic finding, shows as a circular light reflex surrounding the macula. This first becomes apparent at 36 weeks of gestation and is due to changes in the ganglion cell layer. At around 28 weeks, the ganglion cells migrate to the periphery of macula, accumulate there and form a concentric mound. This forms a 'crater-like' appearance at macula, created by a thicker peripheral mound and a thinner central area.

The 'foveal reflex' is the last ophthalmoscopic finding to develop, and can be seen around birth. The explanation of this finding is thinning of inner and outer nuclear layers at fovea, creating again a crater-like formation, known as the 'foveal pit'.

Though the macula may appear ophthalmoscopically normal at birth, but histologically and functionally maturation occurs later in childhood. The most remarkable changes in histology of retina consists of cone diameter, shape of inner and outer parts of cone, and cone density.

At birth, the rod-free region of macula is approximately 1100 μ (micro mm) in size. In next few years, a decrease in the rod-free region of macula occurs due to inward migration of cone nuclei. The rod-free area reaches adult diameter of 700–750 μ by 3 years of life.

Three concomitant changes at macula are directly responsible for improvement of visual acuity with age, and that are:

(1) Differentiation of foveal cone photoreceptors; (2) reduction of rod-free zone; and (3) increase in the cone density.

At birth, the inner cone segments are round and thick, and outer segments are short. The inner and outer segments mature at different rates. By 15 months of age, the outer segments have elongated to almost half the adult size. By 4 years, the outer segments are still 30% shorter than adult size. On the other hand, the inner segments mature faster, assuming the adult architecture by 15 months of age. With thinning of cone receptors, they move closer to each other and become tightly packed. Cone density in the foveal region increases from 18 per 100 μ to 22 per 100 μ by 15 months of age, and further to 30 per 100 μ by 4 years. Adult cone density at fovea is around 42 per 100 μ. Increase in acuity, particularly resolution acuity, parallels the increase in cone density.

Applied aspect: When we discuss the higher levels of vision, we try to understand the phenomena of hypervisual acuity or vernier acuity. The 'cone spacing' in an adult fovea is 2.5 μ or 28 seconds/arc. Beyond this limit, the eye does not function. To discriminate between two fine points or lines, as in hyperacuity, the visual acuity rises to 15–20 seconds/arc, which is beyond the scope of the fovea. Therefore, in such cases, the role of 'visual cortex' comes into play.

At birth, the retinal vasculature is fully developed at the posterior pole. At fourth month of gestation, the vessels are first evident at the disc; by eighth month, the retinal vasculature is complete on the nasal side; but the temporal is fully vascularized several weeks after birth.

Neural Maturation of Vision

INTRODUCTION

The visual cortex comprises of over 50 areas in the human, each with a specified role and distinct physiology, connectivity and cellular morphology. How these individual areas emerge during development, still remains a mystery. Although much research and attention has been given to the early development of the visual cortex, we are far from the knowledge about the mechanisms involved about arealization and maturation of these regions of brain. In recent years, it is beginning to dawn that it is the interplay of the intrinsic (genetic) and extrinsic (afferent connections) cues that are responsible for the maturation of these areas and there is a definite sequence in the maturation of the visual cortex (primary striate cortex or area V1) and the multiple extra-striate/associated areas.

Studies in both humans and non-human primates have begun to highlight the specific neural mechanisms responsible for the development of the visual cortex and the ways by which disturbances in sensory inputs and afferent connections can impact on the normal development. Furthermore, damage to a specific area of visual cortex, such as the 'primary' visual cortex (V1), is a common occurrence as a result of neuro-trauma, hypoxia or disease. But the consequences of such injury differ between the immature and adult brain, with the immature brain showing a higher level of functional resilience and recovery (plasticity). With better techniques for examining specific cortical areas and their connections, we are now able to unravel many riddles responsible for the increased neural plasticity that leads to significant recovery following neural injury in the early part of life. Further advances of our knowledge of the sequences of postnatal development/maturation and plasticity observed during this early phase of life could offer strategies to improve our management following such injuries in the adult brain also.

The visual cortex is subdivided into functionally specialized areas that are distinguishable based on their cytoarchitecture, function, and connectivity. However, the precise time when these multitude areas of visual cortex emerge during development and become functional, is yet to be fully understood.

In last three decades, various modes of investigation have developed which have made possible to delve into the intricacies of brain and understand some of its mysteries. The combinatorial approaches utilizing molecular biology, neuroanatomical studies, use of functional magnetic resonance imaging (fMRI) and proton emission tomography (PET) have dramatically increased our knowledge of the development and functions of these areas of the brain. It is not overemphasis that over 60% of the total brain area is utilized in visual functions, directly or indirectly. Most recently, immunohistochemistry has become an important paradigm in identifying the distribution of distinct cell types in the visual cortical areas.

Work done on primate (Marmoset monkey) brain, which is closest to human, has revealed wonderful facts regarding the topography and complex functions of the visual cortex. It is subdivided into distinct cytoarchitectonic, functional and connected areas, comprising of the 'primary visual cortex' (V1) and numerous extrastriate/associated areas (Fig. 2.1). The innervation of the visual area by the thalamus is also highly segregated with the lateral geniculate nucleus (LGN) specifically innervating area V1 whereas the other thalamic nuclei such as pulvinar innervating the extrastriate middle temporal (MT) area. The discovery and analysis of the visual cortical areas in the human and non-human primates has been a major accomplishment in neuroscience, and has opened new vistas in our understanding of the functions of visual brain.

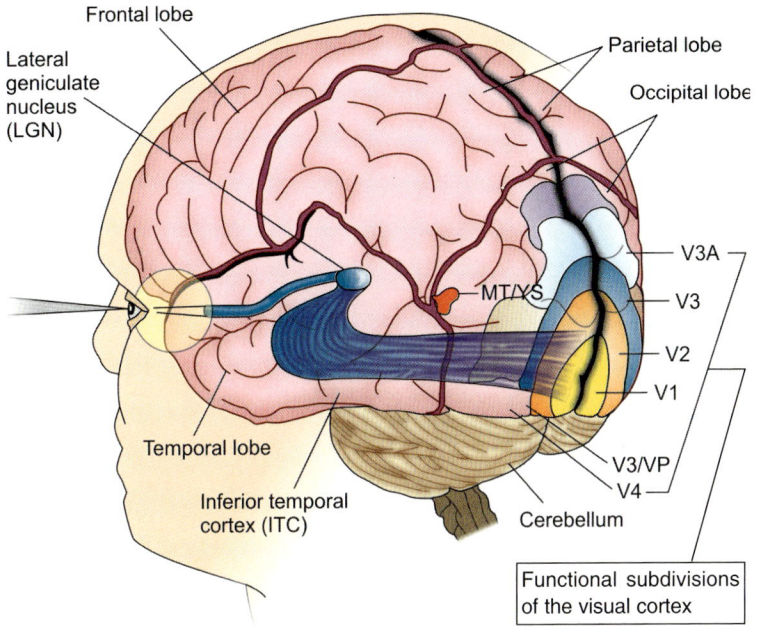

Fig. 2.1: Visual pathways and visual cortical areas

Figure 2.1 is a simplified diagram of the visual pathways that mediate conscious vision from the retina, through the thalamus (LGN) to the primary visual cortex. In addition, there are two disynaptic pathways that bypass V1 and terminate in the middle temporal (MT) area, passing through the cellular layers of LGN and medial portion of the pulvinar (MPL).

Another simplified diagram (Fig. 2.2) depicts the various areas of visual cortex—the primary visual cortex (V1) and the associated visual areas (MT, V2, V3, V4, and so on). Visual information arriving at V1 is relayed to the ventral and dorsal visual processing streams; the dorsal stream diverges from V1 towards the parietal lobe whereas the ventral stream diverges towards the temporal lobe. These streams incorporate the various visual areas that are responsible for processing-specific visual functions. Main visual areas indicated are: V1 (primary

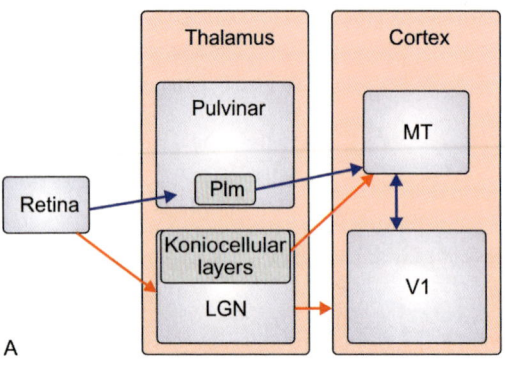

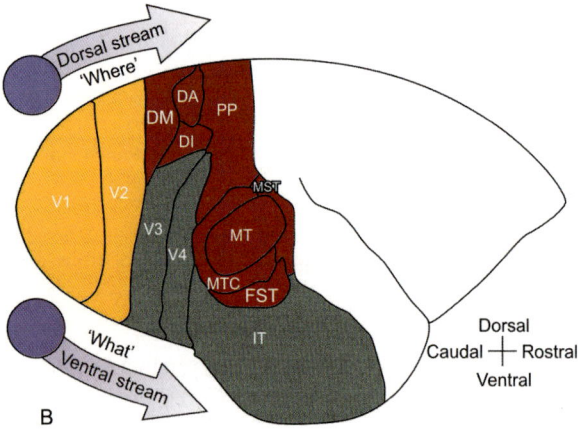

Fig. 2.2: Mapped areas of visual cortex showing dorsal and ventral streams

visual cortex); V2, V3, V4 (extra-striate areas); MT (middle temporal, V5).

It was the earliest works by the German neurologist Brodmann in 1909, on Nissl-substance-stained sections of human brain which demonstrated the 52 cortical areas mosaiced together, defining the primary visual cortex as area 17 and secondary visual cortex as area 18, among other visual areas.

In addition to cytoarchitectural boundaries, retinotopy or visual topography, which describes the spatial organization of neuronal responses to visual stimuli, is used to define the areas 'functionally'. Using specific criteria, it is speculated that each area should comprise a complete map of the visual field. The visual cortical areas such as V1, V2 and MT that have the most organized retinotopy, are referred to as the 'first-order' topography, whereas more complex associated visual areas are referred as 'second-order' topography.

There is yet another commonly accepted but controversial, topographical arrangement of neurovisual connectivity regarding visual processing. This 'two-stream' theory was advocated by Mishkin (1982), in which two parallel visual pathways exist that extend from V1 to either temporal or parietal cortex. According to this hypothesis, there exists a 'dorsal stream' (occipitoparietal) that specializes in spatial/motion vision and a 'ventral stream' (occipitotemporal) that specializes in form/object vision.

Much of data regarding these notions have been obtained from studies of specific lesions in areas of visual cortex (agnosias). For example, lesions in the temporal lobe cause cerebral achromatopsia and loss of form vision in humans, with relative sparing of non-chromatic vision such as motion. It is now well understood that spatial position/motion and colour/form processing is undertaken by separate 'magnocellular' and 'parvocellular' pathways. The projections from magnocellular pathway from the thalamus/lateral geniculate nuclei via the area V1 continues dorsally to area MT and onto the parietal cortex. The parvocellular pathway, in turn, continues from V1 ventrally to V4, and terminates in the inferior temporal cortex. A more recent view of the segregation emphasizes that the dorsal stream governs spatial position and action, whereas the ventral stream governs recognition, and that the 'conscious experience of seeing' is mediated by the ventral stream. But it should be remembered that the acuteness or sharpness of vision, binocular vision and hypervision, is processed in the area V1.

As a matter of fact, so many visual centres are stimulated when the visual input reaches the brain, each centre playing its own part to 'holistically' process what we are seeing and take action appropriately (Fig. 2.3).

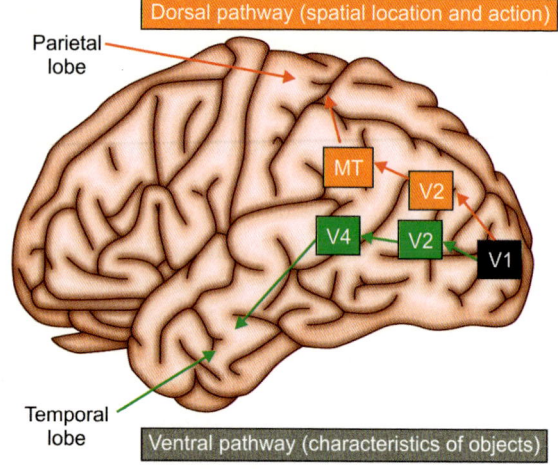

Dorsal pathway (spatial location and action)

Parietal lobe

MT

V2

V4 V2 V1

Temporal lobe

Ventral pathway (characteristics of objects)

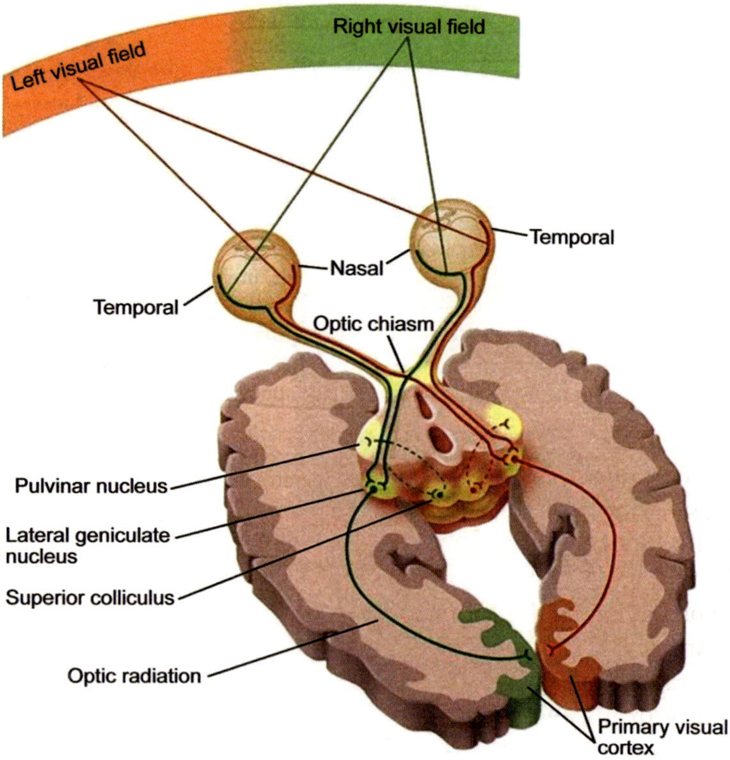

Right visual field

Left visual field

Temporal

Nasal

Temporal

Optic chiasm

Pulvinar nucleus

Lateral geniculate nucleus

Superior colliculus

Optic radiation

Primary visual cortex

Fig. 2.3: Distribution of visual fields

EARLY DEVELOPMENT OF VISUAL CORTICAL AREAS

We have come to know in great deal about the neuronal laminations of the visual cortex, its multi-layered composition, and each lamination comprising of pyramidal and non-pyramidal neurons. More recent studies have now identified the ontogenetic expression/involvement of several proteins in different laminar regions. With the knowledge of multilayered laminated formation of the neurons, researchers are trying to understand the formation of specific cortical areas—the 'mapping of visual cortex'. With the anatomical development/lamination of the brain, there is a considerable 'arealization' which has a unique profile, with certain areas of cortex not maturing well into adolescence. It is this protracted course of 'development/maturation' that has probably been responsible for not able to decipher point-wise development of vision; but at the same time gives us clues about the 'plasticity' of the brain.

The interplay of both molecular (intrinsic) and thalamic (extrinsic) influences (Rakic 1988, O'Leary 1989) is probably responsible for the development of visual cortical areas. The high degree of specificity of 'thalamocortical' connections is essential for the normal processing of sensory information.

Thalamic control: Without doubt, the thalamic innervations of the visual cortex exerts a tremendous influence upon these areas. Although intrinsic factors are more involved in the development of brain in the initial stages, it is the thalamic axons that influence the specific identity and size (arealization) of a particular area. In a study in which bilateral enucleation was performed at mid-gestation in macaque monkeys, retino-thalamic and subsequent thalamocortical connections were lost, and this altered the fate of area V1. The most comprehensive study of human thalamocortical development is by Ivana Kostovic and Milos Judas who retrospectively studied neural connections in more than 500 prenatal brains. In another study of mid-gestational tissues, looking specifically at the development of connections in the human visual system, it was found that human visual connections are partially formed by mid-gestation and undergo further refinement after this period.

The infant human visual brain is quite immature at birth, and consequently vision during the first few weeks of life is characterized by poor acuity, shape and colour perception. Gradually, the visual capacity matures over 8–10 months but some properties reach 'adult-like' only much later, by 9 years of age.

In contrast to this, motion perception is a virtue already present soon after birth, by first couple of weeks. Infants are capable of sensing motion direction soon after birth, and although sensitivity to global-motion (discriminating multiple motions in space) continues to mature till around 7 years of life in humans.

Conventional opinion suggests that a newborn's interaction with the visual world draws circuits in the superior colliculus and thalamic nuclei—but not the lateral geniculate nucleus (LGN). An important evidence that suggests the role of subcortical structures in mediating motion perception in newborns, is based on the 'asymmetry' of optokinetic nystagmus, which is present only in the first few months of life. Brisk 'monocular' reflexes can be elicited in the newborn but only by motion from 'temporal-to-nasal' direction. This early response may be mediated by the colliculus–thalamic subcentres; while the directional sensitivity in the 'nasal-to-temporal' direction, emerging after 10 weeks of life, is mediated by the cortical mechanisms. After approximately 2 months of age, the primary visual pathway through the LGN to the primary visual cortex (V1) becomes the dominant route of visual information. Similarly it was also hypothesized that the visual cortex develops in a hierarchical fashion with higher-order areas developing later, with inputs from previously developed lower cortical areas. The most widely used technique to study the development of visual system in infancy has been visually evoked potential (VEP). However, this does not reveal the isolated or specific cortical areas. Only recently, it has been possible to record fMRI activity in 4–6 months infants who are conscious and look attentively at the visual stimulus

(Biagi et al. 2015). The results were very encouraging and reveal that cortical processing of motion is more mature at this age than previously suggested by other means. The full network of cortical motion areas—including V6, MT (V5) and associated vestibular-visual cortex—is active at this very early age. But the response of area V1 to motion is very immature at this age as compared to other cortical areas. In the humans, area MT receives a strong input from corticocortical connections; but it also receives direct input from LGN and retina via thalamus, both bypass area V1. It is, therefore, hypothesized that early maturation of MT might result from an early inputs from the pulvinar region of thalamus.

Furthermore, it has been suggested by many researchers that area MT is an early maturing visual cortical area and has many properties of sensory primary visual cortex and may play an important role of catalyst in the development and maturation of primary visual cortex. An important and interesting study published nearly 100 years ago, mapping the patterns of myelination (myelination being an indicator of maturation) of the human visual cortex demonstrated that an area referred to as 'field 16' just posterior to the inferior temporal sulcus was one of the very few areas myelinated at birth. The relevance of this finding was recognized in the 1990s when using MRI this area was identified to correspond with extrastriate area MT (Watson et al. 1995). This finding is testimony to the fact that this area MT is an early maturing area.

Recent studies in the marmoset monkey (most comparable visual system to human brain) have further advanced our knowledge of visual system development. Studies have revealed transient nature of a pathway from retina to the pulvinar (thalamus) without involvement of the superior colliculus; which is then pruned during the postnatal period to sparse projections by adulthood. Intraocular injections (anterograde tracers) in marmoset revealed ganglion cell afferents terminated directly to pulvinar region and relayed to MT area in the 'first month of life'. After this time, MT receives most of its visual inputs from the visual cortex, and the thalamic inputs decline in number. The switch in dominance from the 'retinopulvinar–MT' pathway to the 'LGN-V1-MT cortical' pathway, is a major developmental milestone. In the adult, the retinal contribution to the pulvinar is minimal, with the primary driving inputs to all associated visual cortical areas coming from V1.

The above observations have led to the view that the visual pathway in which the pulvinar directly relays retinal inputs to MT, is responsible for early development and maturation of MT. The connectivity between retina, pulvinar and MT is exuberant at birth, and normally regresses dramatically in the first few months of life, after the 'critical period'. Thus, once the retinopulvinar–MT pathway has served its purpose, it becomes surpassed by LGN–V1 pathway.

Environmental factors: Although occurring subsequent to the development of the visual cortex, the formation of specific topographic maps/retinotopy, is also a fundamental part of cortical development.

This experience-based development also acts in synergy with the 'intrinsic' development which provides the final identity to an area and is responsible for the plasticity of the system.

Intrinsic/molecular factors: Although in the past decade, number of genes or 'transcription factors' have been identified, but we are still short of knowledge how many of these molecular machinery actually is essential in the formation of specific areas of visual cortex. Two transcription factors that are believed to be essential for regional development of the cortex are 'Pax 6' and 'Emx 2'. In the human visual cortex, these two genes have been widely implicated in the development of fetal neocortex.

Although the discovery of these genes has opened the possibilities of understanding the role of these genetic transcriptors in the focal patterning of the visual cortex, it does not explain the formation of areas defined by sharp borders of functioning. It is the sharpening of specified functioning areas that is probably the most important feature of corticogenesis.

Another gene identified in 2001, EphA/ephrin, has been found in the areas V1 and V2 during embryonic development of the neocortex in the macaque monkey. (It is to be remembered that these primates resemble most closely in the development of many areas of brain, including the visual cortex.) A number of other ephrins have now been identified and are believed to be critical for regional identification and maturation of the cortex.

FUNCTIONAL MATURATION

Although many researchers feel that the formation of cortical layers and 'arealization' by means of intrinsic and extrinsic influences, as an end point; but in fact, this is beginning of important functional development and maturation of the visual system. As already mentioned, both behavioral and electro-physiological testing in humans have demonstrated that the visual system, particularly the visual cortex, is immature at birth. Although important visual functions gradually emerge during the first year of life, the completion of visual maturation continues until end of childhood, approximately by 9 years of age.

The 'profile' of visual cortical development has intrigued most scientists. We all now know that all the visual cortical areas do not mature at the same stage. But we are still unaware of the precise timing and stages of maturation of individual cortical areas, which may be affected by both intrinsic and extrinsic influences. Studies have established that even normally, there is a significant delay in the development of extrastriate areas as compared to primary cortex. Furthermore, the ventral stream takes a longer time to function than the dorsal stream.

From psychophysical studies in humans, it has been demonstrated a slow development of the perceptual/recognition system, mediated by the ventral stream than the dorsal system that perpetuates the motion/action. Moreover, studies using the fMRI and pattern VEP to examine the face, object/form, selective regions in the ventral temporal cortex of children and adults found that the right fusiform gyrus was not only larger but the response amplitude to 'faces' was significantly higher in the ventral temporal cortex. A glaring example quoted by Fine et al. in 2003, reported a case of patient who was blinded at age of 3 years and subsequently underwent corneal transplants at age of 40 years, and it was demonstrated that although he could perceive motion, but object and face recognition were significantly impaired. Therefore, this proves that the motion pathway was well established and well wired by the time of lesion and more resistant to deprivation; whereas the form processing pathway was still immature and more susceptible to deprivation.

In the developing non-human primate, the acuity of single cell in V1 is found to be worse than expected, based on the density of retinal cone receptors with the acuity of single V1 neuron. It was also found that the 'behavioural acuity' (all round response to stimuli), is quite poor at birth and continues to mature 4 years postnatally, and that the optimal performance is achieved through a refinement in the connections and specific alterations in synaptic architecture of V1.

Binocular vision: Multiple factors are likely to be involved in the maturation of binocular vision. First, is the ability to detect smaller objects and thus the ability to resolve smaller differences in vision between two eyes. Second, is the maturation of 'ocular dominance' columns which appear between 27 and 28 weeks gestation, and mature functionally after eye opening and continues postpartum. Finally, is the refinement of individual neurons in V1 to orientations and inputs from the retina.

Colour vision: Alongside the development of binocular vision and concurrent depth perception, there is development of colour vision also. Surprisingly, human infants actually use colour information to assist in the perception of motion. In a study by Dobkins and Anderson in 2002, showed that 4 months old infants were more capable than adults in discriminating a stimulus that required colour information to detect motion. In other words, coloured objects were more easily detected during motion. Therefore, it was concluded that in infants there was connectivity between motion and colour-processing centres in the brain at this early age, which are pruned/removed in the subsequent postnatal life. This finding also relates to the changes in topography of areas processing motion and form perception in infants as compared to adults.

PLASTICITY OF VISUAL CORTEX

A great deal of our efforts in treating number of congenital and developmental disorders depends upon the capacity of the brain to rejuvenate. Moreover, recuperation from secondary afflictions in the brain also depends upon how and to what extent the central neural system redeems itself. But the exact mechanisms of various areas of the brain, particularly the visual cortical areas, rejuvenates itself, is still shrouded in mystery. Research and speculations, over the last half century, have of course, enriched our knowledge a great deal, and made us wiser regarding many myths; but we are still far from understanding the reorganizations and adjustments the brain tissue makes, better called 'plasticity', to regenerate and revive from inherent and secondary afflictions. We are here, more concerned about the 'developmental plasticity', which has an enormous impact on neuroscience. Our initial understanding regarding this comes from the seminal work of David Hubel and Torsten Weisel (1963), who were honoured with the coveted Nobel Prize in Medicine for their historical work on visual deprivation and recuperation from the insult. They were keen to know whether the response properties in the cells they were studying in adults were innate or were developed later in life by some process similar to learning.

They also wanted to know, if they could alter the response by altering the animals early experience. Though their work was basically done on kittens, but it was later confirmed in non-human primates.

Their experiments were influenced by the observations of Von Senden (1960), that children with congenital cataracts have substantial and often permanent visual defects even after removal of cataracts.

In their earlier experiments, visual deprivation was induced by suturing the eyelid closed. This manipulation did not damage the retina, and the LGN remained responsive after the eyelid was reopened after a few months, but most cortical neurons in area V1 did not respond to stimulation of the deprived eye, although they continued to respond to the non-manipulated eye. They reasoned that during deprivation, the synaptic connectivity must have weakened due to disuse. But after binocular deprivation, they were surprised to note that both cortical neurons remained responsive to both eyes. In another landmark experiment, they tested their 'competition hypothesis', which suggested that the differences in 'amount' of synaptic activity, determined by the visual inputs from retina, determines the strength of connections. Specifically, they raised kittens with artificial strabismus and on examination of cortical neurons noted that the cells responded to either one eye or the other eye, but response was very poor when both eyes were simultaneously simulated, proving loss of function of binocular cells.

To verify these findings, similar experiments were later repeated in macaque monkeys (Hubel et al,1977; Hubel and LeVay, 1980), and almost identical results were achieved. Other researches done in the last two decades have concluded that the remarkably complex and precise connectivity present in the adult visual system arises as a result of an equally extra-ordinary developmental process. Spontaneous as well as stimulus-driven activity fine-tune the connection between neurons in the various visual areas, architecturing the anatomical and physiological properties of neurons and synapses. Similar to pruning, the remodelling of existing synapses has a key role in reorganization of the neural circuitry.

"Synaptic plasticity essentially comprises of number of mechanisms that mediate the activity-dependent and intrinsic modulation of neuronal connections at the level of synapse." The specific reorganization of thalamocortical projections through synaptic remodelling is critical for a number of visual functions. Also equally significant is the remodelling of retino-thalamic connections and synapses which are input-dependent. Similar to the model of learning, inputs originating in the retina of each eye produce step-wise selection of each neuron. Coordinated, identical activity secures synaptic connections and maturation of the neurons, whereas contralateral afferents that transmit weaker and less organized patterns, become less active and are eliminated. This was, in essentiality, the modus operandi for development of amblyopia. However, the classical view of ocular dominance-based plasticity has come under challenge in recent years during which research has demonstrated that other activity-dependent factors are essential for both plasticity and synaptic stability. For example, many molecular factors described above including neurotrophins which promote formation, maturation and stabilization of synapses, have been associated with the development of area V1. Therefore, in human neonates, it is essential to correct disorders which interfere with coordinated and organized inputs from the retina. For example, congenital cataracts should be treated before 6 months of age; strabismus should be treated before 7 years of age. Thus, periods of maturity are different for different circuits in the visual cortex, and constitute critical periods of vulnerability.

Although experience-dependent plasticity primarily pertains to different periods of development, in the adult visual cortex it underpins both perceptual learning and recovery from lesions in the brain. Thus, the study of plasticity in both child and adult has become a major area of research, as it could open new avenues for recovery following visual system damage.

DISTURBANCES OF NORMAL MATURATION

There is significant evidence to suggest that normal cortical maturation is dependent on normal vision.

Effect of monocular or binocular deprivation during cortical maturation can be so severe that it can lead to almost blindness. Disorders such as anisometropia, strabismus and visual deprivation in early age lead to amblyopia. Visual acuity, contrast sensitivity, form recognition, motion recognition, binocularity, etc. are all affected. Visual deprivation has the most severe effect on all these visual functions. Apart from amblyopia, autism, dyslexia, mental retardation, all have severe motion perception deficits, and there is abnormal magnocellular pathway processing.

These are some examples of indirect influences that developmental disorders have on the visual processing and maturation in the visual cortex. However, the specific causes and mechanisms involved are yet to be fully understood. What we have so far resolved is that the phenomenon is likely to involve a cascade of events including molecular, perceptual and physiological factors. In the recent years, great deal of emphasis is being given to the genetic effect on development and maturation. Many genes have been identified as being upregulated and downregulated in the process of non-deprivation and deprivation of the magnocellular and parvo-celluar layers of the LGN. Identification of these genes has opened the possibility of providing potential targets for therapeutic intervention of the disorders.

MECHANISMS OF RECOVERY IN CHILDREN WITH VISUAL CORTICAL LESIONS

It has long been recognized that consequences of injury to the cerebral cortex in the immature brain differ from the consequences of injury in the adult brain. In the immature brain, neurons are more vulnerable to damage and the brain attempts to bypass the damaged or degenerated areas at this early age. Functionally also, the immature brain is more resilient to damage as contrast to mature brain where the consequences are more devastating.

So many of neonatal infections, like encephalitis, meningitis, tuberculosis, are now successfully treated.

Premature infants now survive albeit some perturbations of premature or hypoxic birth problems. Modern management has now made possible for these infants to survive and live. However, the issue still remains how to manage the damage to the 'visual cortex' and the best strategies for recovery of visual functions.

Many reasons have been proposed as how the visual lesions appear to recover. The most obvious reason is that the normal maturation of visual cortex which occurs in children, allows for the 'residual visual potential' to become apparent and active over a period of time. It has been seen that in cases of incomplete removal of visual cortex and optic radiation, some visual recovery after a period of time occurred; which suggests that some specific mechanism of plasticity must be occurring. It must also be noted that a reasonable period of time for recovery is required before significant recovery is observed. This also varies between individuals. Regrettably, a few investigations have been undertaken to study the molecular and physiological recovery at the neonatal level; though we now know that many genes (molecular guidance cues) are expressed at this stage of development.

Muckli et al. in 2009 reported a unique example. A study of a 10-year-old girl who lacked her entire right hemisphere from birth with right microphthalmos, but remarkably had close to normal vision in both hemifields. It was shown that despite having complete loss of right hemisphere, the child's remaining hemisphere has developed maps of both ipsilateral and contralateral visual hemifields. Using *f*MRI showed that in V1 continuous maps of contralateral and ipsilateral hemifilds overlapped each other, whereas in area V2 and V3, small islands of hemifield developed. It was also seen that retinal ganglion cell afferents 'changed' their predetermined crossing pattern at the level of optic chiasma and 'rerouted' to the ipsilateral LGN. Although this is a single case-based analysis, but it opens our eyes to the inordinate capacity and flexible mechanisms involved in topographical map formation during development, which probably involves a number of mechanisms, both innate and extrinsic, in rerouting connections and forming new areas.

Another glaring example was quoted by Reinard Werth in 2006. Two children, aged 19 and 28 months, who suffered from bilateral loss of occipital lobe as a result of a large cyst, had their visual functions tested for visual acuity, fields, contrast sensitivity, eye movements, etc. It was demonstrated that after the loss of area V1 (occipital cortex) in early life, extrastriate areas, such as area MT, are able to mediate many of the visual functions and it was seen that the neurons from LGN targeted the area MT which mediated the visual functions. It was also suggested that in this development, the molecular guidance cues (MGC), which are essentially the neurotransmitters, play a significant role in rerouting the axons from the LGN to other areas of the extrastriate cortex, as they had done in guiding the axons from LGN to the area V1.

In another example, a child of 8 years, who sustained severe injury to left occipital cortex in a road accident, had right homonymous hemianopia with sparing of macula 'extending almost 3.5° to the blind hemifield'.

A pertinent question with all these subjects is whether the observed recovery involves 'new and aberrant' neural connections or whether the 'remaining area of V1' generating over activity.

However, as the main pathway to the visual cortex is destroyed, the recovery of visual functions must arise either from an 'already but inactive alternative' pathway or 'formation of a new' pathway. Using a highly sensitive diffusion tensor imaging, the 8-year-old child showed an alternative pathway from LGN to area MT, bypassing area V1. (It should be remembered that in first 3 months of life, all afferent connections from thalamus go to area MT, which is later pruned and becomes inactive.) In addition, two more major features were observed, i.e. (i) A contralateral pathway from right LGN to left MT area, and (ii) substantial corticocortical connections between area MT bilaterally.

Recent research has laid lot of importance to the area MT (middle temporal) or area V5. The dominant source of visual signals to area MT is direct input from V1. But studies in number of humans have demonstrated that area MT continues to respond to moving stimuli following ablation of V1. Therefore, it proves that alternate thalamocortical connections exist that bypass V1, and are responsible for some of visual functions especially motion perception and global perception. Recent preliminary studies have revealed an increase in 'surface area' of MT on the ipsilateral side, following lesions in area V1 in early life. This emphasizes the increased role of area MT, following loss of primary visual cortex in early life.

In a nutshell, other extrastriate areas of the cortex, especially area MT, develop and provide alternate area of visual cortex to provide some of the visual functions in absence of primary visual cortex. The above mechanisms suggest the plasticity of brain in recovery of visual functions.

SUMMARY

The above mentioned data suggests that the young visual cortex has a greater capacity for recovery and regeneration than the adult. Although recovery of some visual functions has been observed in 'blind sight' patients, but the recovery is far less than an infant brain. Therefore, the next step in the area of regenerative medicine is to harness the mechanisms involved in the maturation of the infantile or neocortex and attempt to recapitulate them in the adult.

We already have some insight into the potential benefit certain molecules have on the development and functional maturation of the cortex as well as the repair/recovery after injury to the visual cortex.

Furthermore, studies have highlighted the role of extra-striate/association areas like area MT has primary cortex like characteristics, which contradicts the textbook opinion on the development of visual cortex. We also now know number of processes involved in the development/maturation of visual cortex, including the role of neurotransmitters/genes, extrinsic and experience-dependent mechanisms. We also know that different areas of visual cortex have different periods of maturation, the importance of 'critical periods' of development and the value of proper visual/retinal inputs.

Finally, we have understood the role of extrastriate areas in taking over some of visual function in cases of injury/damage to the primary visual cortex, by virtue of developing new connections as well as reopening the long lost redundant connections.

Postnatal Development of Visual Functions

One of the most treasured moments in life is when a newborn opens eyes to the world! That vision is very feeble, in shades of grey, but it is the kick start of a vision of the whole universe.

It is important to know that a person has different types of visual functions, which vary in the level of development from person-to-person. We, in normal circumstances, use only visual 'acuity', which is sharpness of vision, to recognize details of any object. Traditionally, visual acuity testing is done by charts having fixed structure of letters or objects, with highest contrast. In our everyday life, objects of various sizes and shapes are viewed in different backgrounds and in different levels of illumination. Therefore, vision encompasses a myriad of visual functions, some fully developed, some underdeveloped. It would be prudent to have a general idea of these functions.

1. *Visual acuity*, or *sharpness of vision*.

2. *Focussing skills:* The ability to maintain clear vision at all distances.

3. *Eye tracking:* The ability of eyes to maintain focus and accurately follow an object. The simplest example includes movement of eyes across a sheet of paper while reading.

4. *Binocular vision:* The ability to use both eyes together to see a single image of an object.

5. *Stereopsis:* To attain depth perception while viewing binocularly.

6. *Colour vision:* The ability to recognize different colours.

7. *Vision of motion:* To gauge accurately the motion of different objects in space.

8. *Form recognition:* This is a higher visual function and is the ability to detect fineness of different parts of an object or differentiate between different objects put together.

9. *Vernier acuity:* This is also known as 'hyperacuity', wherein fine lines can be differentiated. This is a higher visual function requiring involvement of visual centres in the visual cortex.

10. *Visual memory:* To recognize and retain what has been seen and recall what had been seen.

11. *Field of vision:* The ability to see objects in space while fixating at a central point.

For all practical purposes, it is the visual 'acuity' which matters most, and henceforth all references about vision will mainly concern acuity. However, chapters have been included highlighting other virtues of visual performance necessary in day-to-day life. Healthy eyes and good vision play a critical role in how infants and children learn to see!

Let us now consider the various milestones of vision development. This is not only for academic interest, but these milestones enable us to ascertain whether a child's visual development is progressing in a satisfactory manner or not.

At birth, baby's eyes do not focus beyond 8 or 10 inches. Vision in babies undergoes through many changes rapidly in the first few months of life. At birth to a few weeks, babies are very sensitive to bright light, such that their pupils remain constricted to limit light entering their eyes. But the pupillary reaction to light is fully developed and constriction is brisk. This is an important sign for if the pupils are not reacting to light, then a detailed examination is warranted. As a matter of fact, pupillary reaction to light starts eliciting after 32 weeks of gestation, so even in premature babies, light reaction can be elicited.

After 2 weeks, the sensitivity to light becomes less, and the pupils begin to enlarge. The vision improves, but still in shades of grey, and high contrast images in black and white attracts the baby's attention; and this forms our basis for certain tests of vision. More importantly, the most favourite object of attention is the 'human face', and the baby smiles at the sight of mother's face. This gesture is one of the most significant signs of a normal vision at that age. If holding the baby by mother does not show this gesture, then it is doubted whether the baby is seeing or not.

IN INFANTS

From one month onwards, peripheral vision develops faster than central vision.

Vision is still in shades of grey only and visibility still is not more than 8–10 inches. Blinks at bright light.

Most important, pupillary light reflex is brisk, though pupils are constricted.

By one month: The baby begins to recognize 'mother's face' and smiles at the sight of her face. Similar response occurs when familiar human faces come close to the child.

Looks intently at pictures of high contrast—black and white.

Watches the movement of parents closely around the room. Tears appear. Eyes do not move together, appear crossed and may alarm the parents.

By three months: Follows light, faces, and objects. Smiles at familiar faces. Responds by turning face at sound and voices (But this should not be taken as a sign of vision.) This period is sometimes also called 'critical period' of visual development, where the vision is fast developing. Though it should be noted that various visual functions have different periods of maturation, but in this period, if the clarity of image on the fovea is impaired, then a permanent deficit in vision can occur.

By six months: Tries to reach at objects and bats at hanging toys with hands. An early sign of hand–eye coordination. Can stare intently at objects (good, steady fixation). Eyes move together in a coordinated manner. Fixes gaze at objects and follows object movement correctly. (This forms the basis of an important test of vision evaluation in an infant.)

Begins to recognize colours, as fovea is developed. First, red and orange, then blue and yellow.

By eight months: Tries to catch toys with hands. Tries to touch own image in mirror.

Fixes and follows small objects also. Good hand–eye coordination.

By one year: A child can 'detect' small objects. Vision is fairly well developed. Can follow a fast moving object; and stereo-vision begins to develop.

TODDLER

Twelve to twenty-four months: Able to focus on objects far and near. Recognizes faces and objects in books. Can match pictures. Starts playing with toys. Can place blocks in holes—an indication of good hand–eye coordination. Is able to draw a 'straight line—horizontal and vertical'. Can follow a fast moving object, indicating good 'vision of motion'. The visual acuity now reaches to Snellen 6/9.

By three years: Visual acuity now almost 6/6 Snellen. Can recognize shapes, can match or even copy them.

An indication of developing 'recognition acuity'. Can draw a 'square or a circle'. Can put blocks correctly in places. Has the ability to visualize small objects at distances, can identify small crawling insects, and tries to catch them. This also forms the basis of a test for visual acuity.

BETWEEN THREE AND FIVE YEARS

This is the most crucial period of all round development of a child. Not only are the visual functions taking shape, but cognitive and learning capabilities are also developing at a fast pace. Almost 80% of learning, in this period of age, is through vision. Therefore, any visual disability during this period interferes with the mental development of the child.

The child joins the play school, and starts learning and playing with different toys. Can recognize the various objects he/she sees around; with development of visual memory now, a child should be able to recognize and spell out the things seen around. In essence, whatever the child learns in school and around should be able to be reproduced when asked. This again forms a good basis for number of tests developed to evaluate vision of detection, resolution and recognition.

BY FIVE YEARS

Vision is complete by Snellen parameter of 6/6. Good recognition acuity. Can pronounce letters and words, and read sentences correctly. Good 'recall' memory, forming the basis of reproducing what has been learned. Well-developed 'depth perception'.

In a way, the visual acuity and other visual functions like stereopsis, colour vision, contrast sensitivity, etc. have almost reached the adult level; and a child over five years should be able to qualify for a person of normal, well-developed vision.

MILESTONES OF GENERAL DEVELOPMENT

A brief guideline of milestones in a child's development would not be out of place, because many times these milestones go hand-in-hand with the visual development.

From birth to 3 months:
- Smiles at sight of human face.
- Follows moving objects around the room.
- Turns head towards sound.
- Watches intently human faces.

From 3 to 6 months:
- Responds to other people's emotions.
- Enjoys face-to-face play.
- Explores hands and mouth.
- Tries to reach at nearby articles.
- Makes 'babbling' sounds.

From 6 to 12 months:
- Starts recognizing familiar faces.
- Explores surroundings.

- Tries to turn.
- Points at toys.
- Turns to person when hearing own name.
- Responds to 'NO', and simple gestures.

From 1 to 2 years:
- Laughs and gestures.
- Starts crawling, and explores hidden objects.
- Follows simple instructions.
- Detects and tries to reach at moving small objects.
- Tries to imitate simple words.

By 3 years:
- Expresses emotions.
- Plays with toys and tries to assemble blocks, as taught.
- Matches objects and pictures.
- Starts pronouncing words.
- Stands and tries to walk unaided.

By 4 years:
- Starts walking and plays with other children.
- Speaks simple words and letters.
- Highly interested in surroundings, and learns new games.

By 5 years:
- Can speak, sing rhymes, and dance.
- Good hand–eye coordination.
- Can draw a simple diagram, like a circle or square.
- Recognizes things around itself and good recall memory.
- Learning is quick; as learns new words, poetry, etc.

There exists a vide variation in terms of what is considered 'normal' development, affected by variations in genetic, cognitive, physical, cultural, nutritional, educational and environmental factors.

Children reach some or most of the standard milestones at different times from the norm.

Nevertheless, for a healthy child, there is a time framework, where a normal physical, mental, and visual development should take place. Therefore, the significance of knowing the general and visual milestones is that it gives a clue, whether development is progressing normally or not. And thus ensures early intervention to rectify the pitfall.

These developmental norms are called "milestones"—as they define the known pattern of development that children are expected to achieve. Each child develops in a unique way and there may be subtle differences with every child but recognizable deviation from the norm is an ominous sign and helps us to take corrective steps.

Pediatric Eye Examination

This chapter is purposely included to help the pediatric ophthalmologist to learn the basics of how to proceed for examination of a small child.

In a general patients outdoor, the presence of a small child as patient is viewed with some distaste, as most of clinicians are not conversant with the techniques of eye examination of a small child. To be true, ocular examination of a small child requires patience, skill, and some talent. If one has to become proficient as a pediatric ophthalmologist, the person has to train himself to learn the tricks for a smooth and efficient examination in children.

To architect a pediatric clinic, one has to make certain changes in the environment of the clinic. For example, the waiting area should be different than a general patients area, with comfortable sitting and some toys, big and small, which makes the child feel at home rather than a hostile hospital atmosphere. Some institutions arrange a 'play area' where the child can play with during the waiting period. The waiting period should also be not too long, as the child may become sleepy or hungry and would be uncooperative during examination.

It is imperative that the child must be accompanied by the parents, preferably mother. The examination room should be well lighted at the beginning so that the child is not apprehensive to enter. This has an additional benefit, that is, the clinician can 'observe' the child as he/she comes to the doctor.

THE PROCESS OF EXAMINATION

1. *Observation:* Immense amount of information can be had during simple observation of a child. Do not rush to examine the child. Let the child sit comfortably on parents lap for some time. This will give time for the child to adjust to the new surroundings and more importantly, gives time to the clinician to observe the child. Simple observation will reveal a lot of information, viz. the fixation of eyes, any obvious misalignment, nystagmus, etc. The child's behaviour can also be ascertained at this juncture. An irritable child would not co-operate, may not even open eyes and, therefore, the examination may be deferred for other time, or the child may be recalled once he/she has settled. It must be remembered that a sleepy or hungry child will not cooperate and, therefore, it is prudent to let the child have its timely feed and then recalled after an hour or so.

2. *History:* This is most crucial and listened carefully from the parents, since no information can be had from a small child. A very detailed history is not needed as you may lose precious time till the child is cooperative. Relevance of history is the key and unnecessary questions should be avoided. An old adage that the patient is always right does not necessarily apply here. Many a times, the mother/parent is ignorant and may not understand the illness; the social circle around them may not perceive subtle strabismus or nystagmus as a threat to vision. The general thinking that such problems occur frequently in infants and small children and will gradually outgrow with time is deeply prevalent and the parents may not record the time when it was noticed. Sometimes, the parent will casually declare that this problem is present since 'beginning', even it may have arisen just a couple of weeks back. History relating to perinatal birth trauma, hypoxia, febrile illness, or any such birth problem should be specifically asked. At times it is a good idea to ask direct questions, if unnecessarily time is being wasted. A slightly older child may himself narrate certain symptoms and this should be carefully noted. Many children may not

complain of blurry vision—as they have learned to live with it—and appropriate visual test is mandatory. In an older child, the head posture can be observed while he/she is speaking, and other facial anomalies can also be observed at this time.

The problem for which the child has been brought for examination should be asked from the parent or the older child himself. And further queries in that direction should be focused. Whether the ailment is congenital or acquired should be asked and if acquired, then the age of onset. This has a bearing on the prognosis of treatment. If strabismus or nystagmus is observed, then not much information will be gathered from the parents except the frequency or duration of strabismus; but if vision defect is the chief complaint, then parents need to specify whether the child can see lights, respond to gestures, catches small toys, or very small objects, both near and far.

In older children, the child's behaviour in school should be asked, specially for fatigues, headaches, vertigo, sleepiness and regarding any specific complaint which has come from school management. Any neurological deficit should be enquired and the referring physicians' notes be seen. Whether the child is on any medication, should be specifically asked and the type of medication enquired into. Many medications for any neurologic problem or GI problem contain salts that may cause drowsiness and create inattentiveness which may be perceived as vision defect.

The sequence of developmental milestones should be asked and any discrepancy noted. Lastly, the family history is also important. Enquiry should be done of any similar problem in other sibling, or parents or other direct relatives. Previous miscarriages should be enquired.

In short, as much of history possible should be collected in the shortest time possible; as the child may not cooperate for longer period and the actual physical examination become difficult.

PHYSICAL EXAMINATION

Children can be unpredictable, uncooperative, and non-communicative. Children between 1 and 2 years are most difficult to examine. In later ages, they become more playful and communicative. They start knowing toys and listen to your requests.

For infants, the only source of information is their parents and examination during feeding with a bottle makes things easier. Larger, brightly coloured toys are usually used to attract their attention. Noise-making toys are not recommended, as movement of eyes due to 'sound' gives false information.

Infants and children should always be examined when seated on mother's lap, where they feel most comfortable and secure. There should be no hurry to finish the examination, and it is advisable to keep as much distance away as possible. Bright light source should be avoided as it may irritate the child and may close the lids making examination difficult. Children over 2 years are more responsive, and therefore, calling by their name or nickname, makes them feel better. A friendly rapport should be first established with the child before embarking on any manoeuvre. Always begin with 'non-contact' things: Cover test, fixation pattern, red glow, pupillary examination, etc. Many small children get afraid by touch of a stranger, and once they get upset, it is the end of the examination. Allow the parent to show them toys of 'appropriate size', while you watch the eye movements for fixation. Appropriate size means the size of an object recommended for that particular age for testing purpose.

Older children are better to deal with. They can answer regarding their problems and whatever they narrate should be taken note of it. It is again prudent to develop some kind of friendship by asking about their hobbies, their school programme, and about their likes and dislikes, before commencing the physical examination.

External examination: The child's overall appearance and level of alertness can be judged during history taking from parents or child himself. Ocular alignment and position of head should be the first thing noted. The history will guide in which direction the physical examination should proceed including any specific tests required. The position of lids and lid aperture can be evaluated at this time.

Visual acuity assessment—infants and preverbal: After a general idea, the first and foremost step is to assess their visual acuity. Gross visual acuity in infants is mostly tested for fixation and following movements, monocularly. The examiner must know the appropriate size to which the infant may hold attention. For a one month old, the 'human face' is the best target, while a toy of size of 'thumb' suffices for one year infant. Objects (toys) of variable sizes fall in between these two ages. Usually, in infants, slow pursuit movement arises around 4–6 months, but saccadic pursuit is even present before this age. Therefore during evaluation, this has to be kept in mind.

Preverbal children above 1 year of age respond to different varieties of vision testing, which is described in detail in Chapter on Vision Evaluation.

As the child becomes older and reaches the verbal stage, examination and vision assessment becomes simpler, as the child can communicate and also read and write. Snellen prototype visual acuity testing is the standard means of testing.

Fixation: Fixation is tested monocularly and binocularly. In monocular fixation, one assesses whether the patient fixes with the fovea (central) and the quality of fixation. Each eye should be occluded in turn and the smallest possible target, appropriate for that age, that elicits the response should be used. Fixation is assessed for three different functions: Location (central versus eccentric); quality (good versus poor); and duration (maintaining fixation). In day-to-day practice, the dictum CSM is used which denotes 'central, steady and maintained'. Sometimes the word FF is also used for quality maintenance which means 'fix and follow'. Steady, central fixation is a good sign and the vision for that age seems to be normal. Eccentric fixation is an ominous sign and the vision is assumed to be 6/200 or less Snellen. The target should be moved slowly across the visual field to assess the 'quality' of fixation. The target size and distance should be documented. The examiner should be aware of visual milestones in an infant. Newborns have only 'sporadic saccadic' movements with very poor fix and follow pattern. By 6 weeks, infants show some smooth pursuit movements with central fixation and by 8 weeks they have well-developed central and steady fixation with good fix and follow movements. It should be remembered that up to 3–4 months, the smooth pursuit movement (as demonstrated by optokinetic testing) is predominantly temporal to nasal, and this has to be kept in mind when testing for fix and follow movements. One should remember that there is a small subset of patients who have delayed maturation and may not comply to the normal testing; in these cases, it is better to recall after some months, but should show definite CSM by one year of age.

Binocular testing compares the vision of one eye to the other. This test shows fixation 'preference' of one eye and predicts diminished vision or amblyopia in the non-preferred eye. This test has the advantage over monocular testing as even small deficiency of vision can be brought forth as the non-preferred eye may deviate or may not follow coordinated movement along with preferred eye during 'maintenance' of fixation testing. Binocular testing also has the advantage that the vision of one eye may be very low, still the eye may fix monocularly, if the target is very attractive; but the discrepancy will be elicited in binocular testing.

It is important to do monocular testing prior to binocular testing to rule out possibility of bilateral symmetric visual loss.

In patients with straight eyes or microtropia (strabismus less than 10 pd), the fixation preference can be tested using the vertical prism test. In straight eyes, it is impossible to say which eye is fixing. The vertical prism test induces a vertical deviation and, therefore, allows us to examine fixation pattern. Fixation preference testing is a quick and accurate way of knowing fixation preference in cases of amblyopia due to anisometropia, unilateral ptosis, postoperative residual tropias, and other conditions that could cause unilateral amblyopia.

Children who demonstrate poor fixation to above mentioned techniques can be assessed by **OKN drum** or the **Catford drum**. OKN (optokinetic nystagmus) is an involuntary pursuit response to a moving target of high contrast. Since the OKN drum consists of stripes of high contrast, the child is attracted to them even who are disinterested in other targets. The standard response is equivalent to finger counting of 3–6 feet. This is a good test to evaluate fixation as well as vision in infants and younger children.

Other ways of assessing visual function are the preferential looking tests and the PVEP.

Pupillary examination: Newborns have small, miotic pupils which increase in size to about 6–7 mm by teenage and then gradually decrease in size throughout life. It is difficult to elicit direct pupillary response due to extreme miosis and uncontrolled near reflex. Bright light should be avoided as the infant may close the lids; also effort should be made to have the baby fix at a distance toy target to avoid the near reflex. Older children can control their near reflex but still it is wise to let them look at a distance. It is important to identify any afferent pupillary defect, especially in unilateral amblyopias and vision loss due to macular or optic nerve disease. The 'swinging light test' is a good way of knowing the afferent pupillary defects as the 'paradoxical' dilatation to light is an ominous sign of macular or optic nerve disease.

The red reflex: With the induction of high power bimicroscopy and other technologically advanced evaluation methods, the simple evaluation modules have taken a back seat. Nevertheless, in very young children who would be uncooperative, the 'red-reflex' from the fundus has its own place to begin with. It would instantly show any media opacities and gross refractive errors.

Bruckner described a very useful test to determine these anomalies. He used a direct ophthalmoscope in a darkened room and examined the 'red reflex' from the pupil. In case of strabismus, the affected eye would show a brighter reflex with a slightly larger pupil. It has been demonstrated that as small as 5 pd of deviations can be ascertained by this method. An eye with refractive error will show a darker reflex. Amblyopia too can be detected, as when the slit beam is focused on the affected eye, it should fixate on the beam. Non-fixation means that the eye is amblyopic.

Visual fields: As soon as the child begins to fix steadily, say around 2 years, visual fields should be routinely tested. The easiest and quickest way is by 'confrontation method' using an interesting target. Both uniocular and binocular fields should be assessed. If the child resists patching, binocular testing will also yield homonymous defects.

Even in an infant, a fixation target may be used to fixate centrally and then a different attractive target may be brought in the peripheral field. Owing to good saccadic reflex, the infant may suddenly look at the peripheral target once it is brought in the child's field of vision.

Colour vision: Although colour vision is not routinely done in children but may be helpful in decreased vision of uncertain aetiology and constant monitoring in progressive macular disease and optic neuropathies. More often than not, a parent may bring the child to the clinician claiming that he/she confuses between red and green pencil while during drawing for homework. Congenital red-green colour defects are prevalent in about 8–10% of male population and the early it is diagnosed, the better.

The easiest way to determine colour defects is the colour plates. There are two popular types of plate which are helpful in specific situations. The 'Ishihara pseudoisochromatic colour plates' work on the principle of 'colour confusion' and are useful for detection of red-green defects. Most acquired colour defects show in the blue-yellow range, and will be missed on Ishihara plates, unless the defect has extended to red-green range. The advantage of this test is it can be done on illiterate patients as well as children of preverbal age, as only fingers have to be moved on the colour lines.

The other test called 'Richmond pseudoisochromatic plates', previously known as 'Fardy-Rand-Rittler' plates works on the principle of 'colour saturation' and can detect both red-green and blue-yellow defects. Unfortunately, these do not come in illiterate plates and is difficult for young children.

In general, optic nerve disease will more likely show red-green defects, while retinal disease will show blue-yellow defects.

Slit-lamp examination: Slit-lamp in young children is difficult due to obvious reasons. Infants would not open eyes and bright light is not appreciated by infants and young children. As a matter of fact, though hand-held slit-lamps are available but are not worthwhile as a good means of examination. In small children, examination under general anaesthesia is the best way for microscopic as well as indirect ophthalmoscopic examination.

Refractive errors: Determination of refractive errors is most important in all examinations. Not only knowing refractive error in cases of strabismus is mandatory, but for a host of complaints it is wise to do a cycloplegic test for refractive errors. The clinician may be surprised to detect refractive errors in so many vague complaints by children. It should be remembered that the adequacy of cycloplegia, not dilatation, is important. Also the type of cycloplegic used according to age, and the colour of iris should be kept in mind. The details of these drugs are listed in the Chapter 6 on Management of Refractive Errors.

Fundus examination: Last but not the least, an adequate fundus examination is imperative for children. For most patients, visualization of posterior pole (optic disc and macula) usually suffices. For detailed peripheral examination, anaesthesia is usually required. Infants below 1 year can be sedated and examination can be performed with slightly dim light. Young children around 2 years may not get sedated, and anaesthesia may be required. Children who are older than 3 years are more cooperative and periphery can be examined in sitting position by explaining them the procedure, which is more acceptable to the child.

Assessment of Visual Acuity

INTRODUCTION

Visual acuity means acuteness or 'sharpness' of vision, i.e. the ability to perceive small details.

Though 'vision', in true sense, relates to a number of virtues which are used to perceive and comprehend the world around us (which have been discussed in the Chapter on Development of Vision), but 'visual acuity' is the most important virtue of sight.

The testing of vision in infants and children has been treated seperately from testing of adults because children cannot be tested with the same techniques and materials as in adults. In addition, the course of visual and cognitive development must be taken into account in evaluation of vision at these early ages.

Moreover, special techniques are to be used in assessing visual abilities in small children. An important aspect is that after a particular period in age, the vision remains constant throughout life, but in infants and children, visual abilities are changing rapidly and thus tests and techniques for assessment of vision also change accordingly. Furthermore, certain hyper-acuity abilities continue to develop well into teen age and their assessment is also important for comprehensive visual examination.

A major difficulty in assessing vision in infants is that they cannot be tested with the standard tools that are used in adults. Secondly, studies have shown that vision in infants and children is far inferior to adults. In both normal and visually-at-risk infants, the time course of measured improvement for vision depends on both the assessment technique used and the aspect of vision being tested. Finally, assessment of vision is complicated by the fact that evidence of normal and abnormal visual at one age is not necessarily of what the visual status will be at later age. That is, visual status in infancy is highly plastic and can be intercepted or modified by external or internal environmental factors. Because of the immaturity of infant's visual system and the dynamic nature of visual development especially in first year of life, any system of visual examination in infants must recognize two important points. First, the results of vision assessment must be compared with available normative data from infants of 'same age' and having been tested with the same method. Secondly, results of visual assessment conducted during infancy should not be followed in a predictive way in assessment at later ages. An infant whose vision appears normal in early life, may later show visual impairment, if the visual system fails to show the normative line of development due to any reason. Similarly, some infants who appear visually impaired early in life, show normal responses later. It should be also noted that though the accuracy of tests in infant age group is doubtful, but they are sufficient for broad assessment of vision.

In preschool age, that is around 3–4 years of age, the cognitive abilities have sufficiently developed so that more accurate tests of quantitative nature can be implemented. In general, children of normal intelligence with normal milestones development who have reached 5 years and above, can be tested with same methods as adults. But still their results are typically lower than those of adults. In addition, it is advisable when testing school-age children to use modified procedures that permit the child to respond in a non-verbal manner.

The most prevalent means of measuring visual acuity is by letter chart in children (who can read) as in adults, which was introduced by Snellen and Donders in 1862, developed at the Eye Hospital in Utrecht in Netherlands. Though many variants have subsequently been developed for assessing visual acuity in persons who are literate and illiterate, the principle remains the same; and we will maintain the Snellen letter chart version as prototype in all future discussions.

Before we embark on the study of vision charts and their methodology in children, first let us understand the mathematics of visual acuity in general.

Visiual acuity measurement by the Snellen method is so common and so easy to apprehend, that it has become the gold standard for testing visual acuity. "Snellen acuity measures a fixed size of letters or optotypes in high contrast setting of black and white under standard fixed conditions of illumination".

But in our everyday life, there are objects small and large, have different contrasts, or are presented in busier backgrounds and at different levels of illumination. In all these situations, visual acuity will differ.

Nevertheless, for most practical purposes, the visual acuity testing, based on the Snellen's principles, remains a good indicator of our vision. Moreover, almost all types of vision tests, used for detecting the 'Resolution' visual acuity in children, are based on Snellen principle, hence we have to understand its methodology in detail.

Since the value of visual acuity compares a subject's performance to the performance of a standard eye, 'that' standard has to be defined. Snellen chose to define it as "the ability to recognize his letters when they subtend a visual angle of 5 minutes of an arc at the eye, and the details of that letter when they subtend an angle of 1 minute of arc". The letters were termed as 'optotypes', as they were specific, conforming to the 5 by 5 minute grid, with each 'part' of the letter conforming to 1 by 1 minute graticule. Later, as the Snellen optotypes had some discrepancies, similar new optotypes were later introduced by Louise Sloan. This will be discussed later.

Most people are familiar with the notation of visual acuity as a 'fraction' but a few understand what it actually means. Keeping in mind the Snellen principle of vision, if a person needs twice as large or twice as close a letter, as those needed by a standard eye, then that person's vision is said to be 'half' of normal. If the letters needed are five times larger, then the person's visual acuity (VA) is 1/5th of normal; if ten times larger is needed, then VA is 1/10th of normal, and so on. The values of these fractions can be expressed in different ways, e.g. if 20/20 (6/6) is a normal VA, then 20/40 (6/12) is half the normal; 20/100 is one/fifth of normal; and 20/200 is one/tenth of the normal. Snellen expressed this in the well-known formula: VA= D/M—Viewing distance (meters)/Letter size (in metric units). Snellen insisted that the numerator of this fraction should indicate the 'viewing distance', which should remain constant; while the letter size should change, in denominator, which would indicate his vision at that distance. To extrapolate this into simple terms, if the same letter viewed at 20 ft (6 meters) has to be seen clearly from 200 feet or 60 metres, then it has to be 'ten' times larger. And at all distances, the visual angle of five minutes is maintained, in order to view an object distinctly (Fig. 5.1). But there are examples where an indivisual can perceive an object which subtends even smaller than 5 minutes of arc angle at the fovea. This, in metric terms, is expressed as vision of 6/5 or 6/4., explained as a person can perceive an object at 6 meters which others perceive at 5 or 4 metres!

The numerator fraction is different in different countries, i.e. in USA, feet is used whereas in most countries, metric system is used. Moreover, the viewing distance, i.e. the numerator is also modified according to the convenience. With this change in viewing distance, the size of the letters is correspondingly altered.

Interestingly, the near vision chart optotypes size is also altered for near vision testing, but conforming to the Snellen

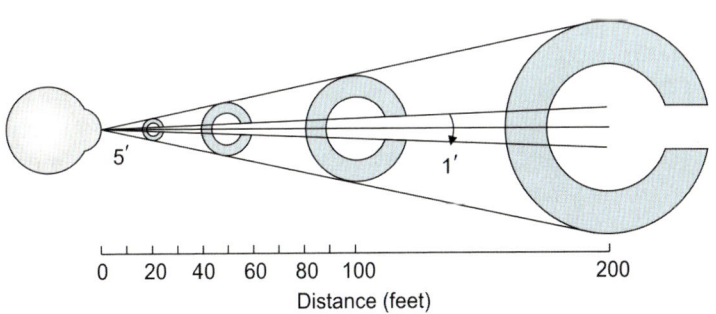

Fig. 5.1: The figure is self-explanatory to understand that to view clearly any object at near or far, the size will correspondingly change albeit, conforming to rule of the 5' (min of arc) for the whole object and 1' (min. of arc) for the details

principle of visual angle of 5 minutes and 1 minute. It should be noted here that at the time of Snellen, the physiological limits of vision were not thoroughly studied and it is only in late 20th century, that we have come to know that a person can discern fine lines and details of an object which subtend an angle of 'less' than one minute-of-arc. This is known as 'hyper-acuity' where the visual acuity can identify objects subtending an visual angle of even 20–30 'seconds-of-arc.'

Louise Sloan further strengthened the concept of Snellen visual angle by putting a 'unit' mark. Thus 'one Sloan unit' or '1-M unit' subtends an angle of 5 minutes at the fovea at a distance of one metre.

Interestingly, 1-M unit happens to be the size of an average news print!

THE PHILOSOPHY OF MEASUREMENT

Since Snellen letter or optotype charts contain discrete letters/optotypes, the measurement accuracy will depend upon the increment of letter size of each line. Most traditional charts have irregular increment of letter sizes, as did the original Snellen charts.

For example, from 6/5 to 6/6 is 33% increase; from 6/6 to 6/9 is 25% increase, but from 6/36 to 6/60, it is 100% increase. It was soon realized that equal increment would be more desirable. The first chart with such a sequence was proposed by John Green of St. Louis in USA in 1868. He proposed a geometric (logarithmic) sequence, e.g. 1.0, 1.25, 1.5, 2.0, 3.0, 4.0, 5.0, 6.0, etc. This sequence of increment in letter size later became to be known as 'perfect numbers'. Unfortunately, Green was far ahead of his time, his proposal was soon forgotten and it took more than a century until this sequence was accepted generally as a standard visual acuity measurement.

Fig. 5.1 is self-explanatory to understand that to view clearly any object at near or far, the size will correspondingly change albeit, conforming to rule of the 5' (min of arc) for the whole object and 1' (min. of arc) for the details.

FUNCTIONAL APPLICATION OF VISUAL ACUITY (VA)

Traditional VA values are well suited for calculations about letter size, magnification and viewing distance. For calculations and comparisons of functional effect of different acuity levels, this geometric sequence cannot be relied upon for number of reasons: Firstly, the increment in size of letters in different lines is not uniform; secondly, the number of letters in each line is not equal, which hinders the exact 'quantification' of vision. For example, in a five-letter line, if three letters are read, it is assumed that the line is read. But in a three-letter line, what notation should be followed? Lastly, the distance between the lines is also not equal, and thus reading in small letter lines may result in some sort of crowding phenomena. Therefore, we need a scale, where all the parameters remain constant.

We, as clinicians, have long used the expression that visual acuity has changed by certain 'number of lines'. This expression is only valid, if the stepwise increment between the lines are equal, as stated above. Equal steps imply a logarithmic progression. Taking the logarithm of each value, converts the geometric progression of letter size to a linear scale of functioning. Two linear scales are available:

1. **The LogMAR scale**, which uses the logarithm directly. In the context of physiologic optics, MAR is interpreted as 'Minimum Angle of Resolution', whereas in a functional context, it is 'MAgnification Requirement'. Although, LogMAR acuity is often presented as measure of acuity, it is actually a measure of the 'acuity loss'. A logMAR value of '0' indicates 'no loss' in vision, a visual acuity of 6/6. A vision better than 6/6 will then be represented by negative (minus) logMAR values. The scale, thus, consists of lines from '0' to '1', with each line indicating 0.1, 0.2, 0.3, and so on as a measure. The advantage of this system is that it also measures the 'partial' gain or loss of acuity; meaning that each single letter has a value of 0.02, and five-letter line would then be represented by 0.1. Thus if 3 letters are read in a line, the visual acuity will be indicated as 0.06 of that line. For example, if a line of 0.2 is read fully and only 2 letters of next line (0.1) are read, then VA will be 0.1/0.04. This entails that

in review situations, if the person's vision improves by further 2 letters (VA now 0.1/0.08) and an improvement of 2 more letters is appreciated. For further standardization, the logMAR system is incorporated in the ETDRS charts.

2. The second scale is the **'Visual Acuity Score'**, VAS system. It is the inverse of the LogMAR system. Though it serves the same purpose, it is more intuitive, as it avoids the decimal values and is more understandable as higher values indicate better vision. Like ETDRS charts, with 5 letters in each line, the VAS increases by 1 (one) point for each letter read correctly (5 points for each line).

   The scale is represented in square brackets, as 100=6/6 and 50=6/60. Thus, with each line indicating 5 points, from 50 (6/60) to 100 (6/6), would then be 10 lines in between.

   But this system is rarely used in practice.

> *Points to note* ....
>
> When assessing visual acuity certain standards have to be looked into, e.g. corrected refractive error, pupil size, illumination, time of exposure of the target, area of retina stimulated, adaptation state of the eye, eye movements. These are self-explanatory and need no further description.

VISUAL ACUITY IN CHILDREN

Extrapolating the above mentioned visual acuity measurements in children, a number of discrepancies arise. All the above discussion and parameters of visual acuity assessment apply to an adult vision, where 'recognition acuity'/'resolution acuity' has fully developed. Infants and small children do not have recognition acuity, only primitive 'detection' ability. In the era of Snellen, pediatric vision examination did not exist or was very limited. It was only in the late 20th century, with the development of neuroscience and child psychology, that vision examination in small children came into existence. With the colossal economic loss and emotional burden of a blind child and its psychological repercussions, serious thoughts began to emerge regarding recognition of a child's visual status. Since Snellen optotypes or its variants were not applicable in small children, assessment of vision was mainly qualitative and arbitrary.

The long, painstaking research of Dr Teller, Dr Gardiner and Dr Sheriden opened new vistas in evaluation of visual status in small children.

The development of electrophysiological techniques, and other psychological tests have enabled us to determine vision even in infants, quantitatively and with remarkable accuracy.

Eventually, more tests and methods to determine visual acuity in toddlers and preverbal children came into existence. Most of these are reproduced in different ways but are helpful in different situations. With expansion of our knowledge in the development of the neurovisual system, better and reliable visual assessment techniques were developed by several researchers, taking cognizance of the age-related maturation of the neurovisual system.

Proper and correct evaluation of the visual status of a small child is one of the most significant part of pediatric ophthalmology.

Somewhere along this chapter, a brief introduction of some revered scientists has been given, as a tribute, to those who contributed brilliantly to the development of vision tests in children.

GENERAL CONSIDERATIONS

Evaluation of vision in children is an art and requires skill and patience. Correct assessment of visual acuity is the first step to guide to evaluate any visual defect. Further, it is the most important guide to assess the improvement during follow-ups.

Vision examination in small children requires special tasks, special equipment, special training, and good judgement. A small child may be attentive for a very short time and then becomes unresponsive. Also repeated visits may be required, depending upon the mood of the child.

Certain variables must be kept in mind during visual acuity testing, viz. the child should not be sleepy; well fed; in good mood. The parents must accompany the child. Many a times, some relative brings the child, with whom the child may not be very comfortable. It is important that the child must feel fully secure and comfortable during examination. The child must be seated in the mother's lap, where he/she feels most secure. Some hospitals have special play area for children, where they can relax and play, before being called in for testing.

Furthermore, the environment of the examination room should be child friendly, the child should feel interested in the test, and understand the test being used.

The test should be explained in the language the child understands, as far as possible, to a preverbal or verbal child. If you only talk to the mother, the child will loose interest. If the child is sick, hungry, or sleepy, postpone the evaluation. It may sometimes be necessary to explain the test to the mother and let her conduct the test, while you observe the child's response. As will be highlighted later in this chapter, different, age related sized 'toys' are used to get best results. But caution should be excercised not to use sound producing objects, as visual attention is masked by sound attention.

The following parameters should apply to the tests being employed.
1. Test should attract the child.
2. Should be child friendly.
3. Reproducible
4. Reasonably accurate
5. Should be age-matched.

Decades of research and clinical experience by psychologists, pediatricians and ophthalmic experts have been able to develop number of tests, which have stood the test of time, and have helped us to determine, with reasonable accuracy, the vision of infants and children.

No test, however, is exact and gives hundred percent correct value. Most of the tests which have evolved over the time are age specific and they are so programmed that a child of a particular age will respond appropriately to that test. These tests take into consideration the psychology and age-related visual maturation of the infant and child.

Unfortunately, most of the centres neither have the standardized procedures nor the know how to perform these tests. Nevertheless, if one single test is mastered and performed properly, it gives ample information of the visual status of the child.

Many of these tests overlap. In other words, the same test is performed in a different way or using different subjects. Many of them overlap in different age groups, but are authentic as the child's visual milestones may not follow a standard pattern.

'Reproducibility' of the result is perhaps the key to a successful visual examination, and it is a measure of a child's subjective or 'everyday' visual competence. Most of these tests, especially in infants and small children, require skill and special training to perform. These tests were devised keeping in mind the development and quality of vision at different ages. Some of these tests may not give accurate quantitative analysis of visual acuity, but still give us a fairly good result to work on.

As already stated, vision is not only 'visual acuity'. As the neurovisual system matures, number of more sophisticated visual functions develop and are extremely useful in our everyday life. These will be dealt later in this chapter.

Developmentally, visual acuity may be classified as: (1) Detection, (2) Recognition, and (3) Resolution.

These basically denote the improvement in visual acuity as the level of visual maturation improves.

Detection acuity is the most basic of vision and begins presenting a week after birth. The fovea and the visual cortex are so underdeveloped that an infant sees everything in shades of grey and cannot identify beyond 10–12 inches. The 'human face' is the best object an infant can identify and appreciates it with a 'smile' when a human face is presented. This is because the first thing a newborn sees is the 'mother's face' and correlates every face with it. This is so convincing, that it is used as a strong measure of visual acuity in a neonate.

By 4–6 weeks, an infant begins to detect certain 'patterns', the most simple being 'gratings' of high contrast, i.e. black and white. Gratings are black and white bands, alternating with each other. Since the visual acuity is still in shades of grey, this is the most 'fundamental' indication of vision development. Though this is only a 'qualitative' assessment, some gross idea of the level of visual acuity can be had by decreasing the 'width' of the black stripes, which are presented to the infant. It is to be remembered that only 'high contrast' can be identified by the infant up to 4–6 months of age; so it is basically the black stripes or gratings which the infant is identifying against the 'white background'. The vision in an infant at birth, as deduced, by these tests, is less than 6/200.

As the infant grows, the neurovisual system matures; the child starts recognizing the shapes and contours of objects and also the colours. The development of fovea is complete in most part, by 6 months of age, an important milestone to be kept in mind; and, therefore, an infant starts recognizing colours after this age.

It is to be noted, that up to 1 year of age, the visual system matures very rapidly and vision develops at a great pace. As mentioned in Chapter on Vision Development, this is a crucial period, also called the 'critical period', and any impediment in the clarity of vision occurring during this period leaves a permanent disability in vision. Though there are different 'critical periods' for different types of vision, but birth to 3 months and then up to 1 year are most significant in visual development. By 1 year of age, the visual acuity has supposedly reached around 6/12, but is difficult to assess.

More than the estimation of visual acuity by standard methods, a child's 'expressions' speak a great deal of its visual status.

Till the child does not speak, i.e. up to 2½ to 3 years of age, called the Toddler period, visual acuity status can be assessed only indirectly. Though there are a battery of tests available, they all contribute to a 'fairly' good assessment but not 'accurate' assessment of visual acuity.

Nevertheless, these tests, if judiciously performed, are a good indication of vision up to a 'preverbal' age of the child.

After 3 or 4 years of age, the child begins to speak, and with visual memory well developed, can reproduce written letters, objects and various forms. This is the fully developed 'recognition acuity', and remains throughout life.

Based on the scientific knowledge of the various levels of visual development and maturation, different tests have been devised which are 'age specific'. They are used within a 'range of age period', and may overlap.

Therefore, tests devised conform to the following age groups:

1. Infants—up to 1 year of age.
2. Toddler—1 to 3 years of age.
3. Preverbal—3 to 5 years of age.
4. Verbal—after 5 years of age.

Let us now examine each of the age-related tests.

VISION EXAMINATION IN INFANTS

An infant is assumed up to 1 year of age. This period is the most significant and most difficult in terms of assessing the visual acuity.

a. *Pupillary reflex:* In a small baby, this is perhaps the simplest and most valuable indication of vision. Pupillary reflex, both direct and consensual is well developed at birth, and can be elicited at 32 weeks of gestation. The only care to be taken is that infant's pupil is miotic, the constriction is subtle and it is better to examine the reflex with room lights off.

Stiles-Crawford effect: It would not be out-of-place, to mention an observation noted by the scientists. The observation mentions that pencils of light entering the eye 'obliquely' are a less effective stimuli as compared to light entering centrally. This is not due to any aberrations in cornea, but due to orientation of receptors in the retina. This is known as 'stiles-crawford effect' and has relevance in precisely assessing the afferent pupillary reflexes. Therefore, in an already small pupil, subtle movement of pupil in assessing the afferent pupillary reflex is of great significance.

b. *Observation:* Devote some time to carefully observe the movements of eyes. Wandering eye movements is an ominous sign that the infant is not seeing. Also the position of eyes can be determined. Obvious misallignment of one eye, heralds strabismus, and an indication of vision defect.

c. *Eye contact:* 'Eye contact' is the most powerful mode of establishing communication in humans. From a few days after birth, the baby begins to look at known faces, especially mother's face. The baby looks intently at faces and maintains 'eye contact' for fairly long time. This is an important paradigm in assessing vision quality in an infant.

d. *CSM:* CSM is an acronym and stands for the child's gaze or child's visual attention being central, steady and maintained. The procedure is that a specific age-related target is presented to the child uniocularly. The object should not make any noise and should be under sufficient illumination.With one eye occluded (by any way), the target is shown from a distance of around 40 cm or half meter. The eye under observation is noticed. The infant should stare at the object intently, eyes being straight and pointing to the object. This shows foveal fixation. The target object is then slowly moved from one side to other, and the eye should follow the object. This proves that the fixation is 'steady' and 'maintained'.

Each eye is examined separately in this manner and the test gives a fairly reliable status of the vision in each eye. The difficulty is that the child should get interested in the target he/she is looking at, otherwise the child will lose interest and move the eye haphazardly.

Many a times, the child may not allow to occlude one eye, in which case no occluder should be used as the child may be intimidated. In such situation, the hand may be used as an occluder, that too from a distance.

To assess the fixation pattern, a specific target is selected to which the child's gaze is attracted. It is to be remembered that there are 'age-specific' size fixation targets. To recapitulate, from one month to six months, a child can fixate the size of a human face to a small toy. By end of first year of life, a target of 'thumb nail' size is enough to attract attention. Various types of targets can be used, like dolls, animals, monkey faces—the more fascinating the target, the more it is liable to attract attention. (Figs 5.2 and 5.3).

If the child 'resists' occlusion of any eye, then it is a sign that the eye under occlusion is the seeing eye and the child tries to remove the occluder when the seeing eye is occluded.

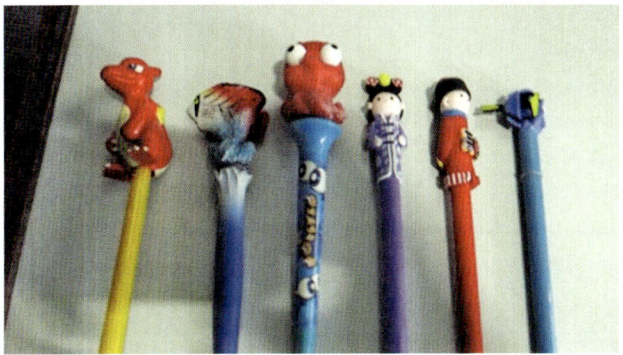

Fig. 5.2: Target of thumbnail size

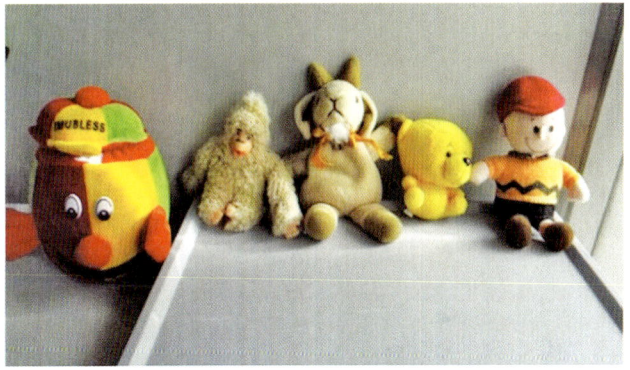

Fig. 5.3: Larger target for 3 to 6 months infant

In such a situation, the manuevre should be repeated number of times to be certain of the reaction from the child. In case of doubt, it is prudent to further investigate.

e. *Dolls eye manoeuvre:* This is to elicit the vestibulo-ocular reflex (VOR). The head of infant is turned to one side and movement of eyes is observed. The eyes move in opposite direction to the movement of head. This shows an intact vestibulo-ocular motor pathway and intact brainstem pathway of oculomotor nucleus to the eyes, and proves the stability of central gaze fixation to the target, when the head moves to the other side.

f. *Visually evoked potential (VEP):* **This is a great test which** electrophysiologically evaluates the visual system right from macula to the visual cortex. Suitable electrodes are placed on different positions on the head, and vision is stimulated by presenting the retina with an illuminated pattern stimulus. The electric response is determined on a graph.

The test requires special equipment and is a sensitive test. It is usually done where the fundus is found to be normal and no refractive error is detected, but where fixation is defective and visual status of infant is thought to be subnormal. As already described in Chapter on Development of Vision, VEP has proved to corroborate visual status extremely reliably with the development of vision.

VEP studies describe a more rapid rate of visual development. With VEP, there is a steady but more fast improvement in visual acuity from 20/400 (6/120) scale in newborns to 20/20, i.e. 6/6 by 10 months of life. The vast difference between the values registered by VEP and PLT has been the subject of much debate. VEP has the theoretical advantage that it does not require a motor response from the child—which may be not always dependable—and, therefore, is more accurate and sensitive. VEP measures the response from the primary visual cortex (area V1); but in factuality, visual perception requires involvement of 'more' areas than V1 only, and, therefore, may overestimate the visual response.

g. *Fundus examination and refraction:* **Needless to say, these are** an integral part of examination for the doubtful vision. Macula and fovea are well developed by 6 months of age, though the 'foveal pit reflex' may not be so pronounced. In case of a normal looking fundus and no refractive error (done under deep sedation or general anaesthesia with proper cycloplegia), if vision status is under doubt, the child should be subjected to an electrophysiological examination.

Two more tests, which are applied to the toddler group, are also used in the infants, around the age of 1 year. They are the Teller's acuity cards and Catford drum. They will be subsequently discussed in the toddler group.

VISION ASSESSMENT IN A TODDLER

Optokinetic Nystagmus

This is a slow pursuit movement of eyes following an object moving across the visual field, from one side to another. This is followed by a saccadic recovery to the normal position. The test is a measure of detection acuity.

A simple, easy and quick way of eliciting an optokinetic reflex is by a Catford drum (Fig. 5.4).

GV Catford and A Oliver invented the drum test way back in 1970s. The drum has a white background with vertical black stripes, and is slowly rotated in one direction. As the black stripe comes into view with the movement of drum, the eyes follow

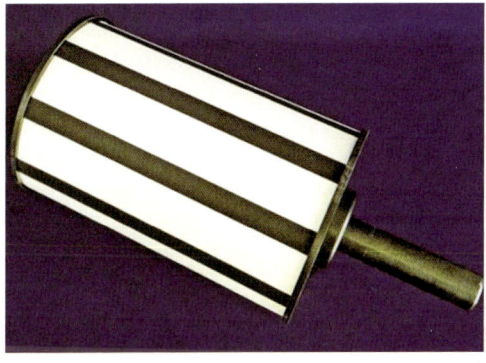

- It is a detection acuity test.
- It is useful in infants and preschool children.
- In this test, the children is made to observe an oscillating drum with black dots of varying sizes.
- The smallest dot that evokes pendulat eye movements denotes the level of visual acuity

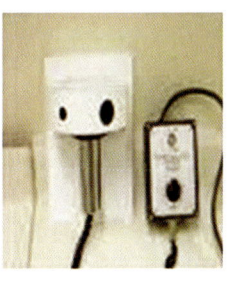

Fig. 5.4: Catford drum test for toddlers

it; and abruptly moves back to the original position as the stripe disappears.

With the rotation of the drum, the eyes resume the following movement as another stripe comes in the visiual field. The drum can be rotated manually or can be motorized. With the latter device, the rotation is more controlled and the speed can be varied. If the drum is rotated at a certain speed, the eyes move more quickly and a state of nystagmus can be demonstrated.

Instead of a stripe, a 'black dot' can be used on the Catford drum. The thinnest stripe or the smallest dot, which still can elicit the reflex, gives the measure of the visual acuity. It should also be remembered that in infants below 3 months of age, the pursuit movement is from temporal to nasal and later becomes nasal to temporal or both ways. Therefore, in testing below 3 months, this point should be kept in mind. Practically, OKN is not advisable before 3–4 months because of unsteady ocular fixation.

The dot or the stripe conforms to the size of the Snellen opto-type, presenting an angle of 5 min at the fovea. The size varies from 6/60 to 6/6 of Snellen optotype. The smallest size which continues to elicit the the reflex, gives the measure of vision.

Dot Acuity Test

The Dot visual acuity test is based on the concept as the smallest black dot that a child can view and 'point out to or touch' it. By varying the size of the dot, visual acuity from 6/200 to 6/6 can be ascertained in a fairly accurate way (Fig. 5.5).

Preferential Looking Tests (Forced Preferential Looking Tests)

'Preferential looking' tests are a gold standard to assess visual acuity in infants and children alike to a reasonable accurate level. These are by far the most popular and reliable tests for assessing the visual acuity from 1 to 3 years of age.

Using PL testing, VA of newborn is estimated to be around 6/200 (30 minutes of arc).

A rapid improvement to 6/60 occurs by 3–4 months, followed by gradual but steady improvement to 6/12 level by

Toddlers (14 months– 2½ years)	
1. Hundred and thousand sweet test 2. The Cardiff acuity test 3. Dot visual acuity testing.	• Black dots on white background. • Touch a black dot • Test dist.—25 cm • VA—20/800 to 20/20 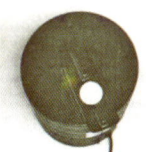

Fig. 5.5: Dot acuity test for toddlers

end of 1 year age. By 3–4 years of age, the VA reaches to 6/6 Snellen. There may be a small variation as some children show VA of 6/6 by 5 years of age.

There are two tests in this category: The Teller Acuity Cards and the Cardiff Vanishing Optotypes. Both are based on the principle that a child 'prefers' to look at an object or a design, rather than a blank surface, when both are simultaneously presented.

Teller Acuity Cards

The test was introduced by **Dr Davida Young Teller** (1938–2011). She was professor of child psychology at the University of Washington, USA.

Dr Teller researched on quantitative behavioural studies of vision in adults and development of vision in infants, in particular. In her career, she created a way to prove how a baby's sight develops and found that infants see mostly 'high contrast' combinations. She found that an infant can recognise, in early life, only 'patterns' of high contrast, i.e. black and white. The pattern of black and white 'stripes', alternating with each other, are the best way to evaluate the vision of an infant and toddlers. Thus, the 'grating acuity' concept is the direct result of her work.

The importance of Dr Teller's work in the field of visual development is widely recognized. She recieved many awards and honours in her illustrious career.

Grating module is an important means of assessing the visual acuity in infants and toddlers. As the resolution power is very weak, infants can detect the black and white bands and 'prefers' to look at the bands rather than a plain sheet. The test can also give a quantitative result to some extent, depending how attentive the child was.

The gratings or bands have a fixed parameter. One black and one white band in one degree is called 'one cycle per degree'. As per norms, an infant of 6 months old can detect up to 5 cy/degree (6 min/arc). By 5 years of age, a child reaches almost adult levels of 30 cy/degree (1 min/arc) or 6/6 Snellen. This means that an infant gets attracted when gratings of 5 cycle in one degree is presented to it. Beyond this limit, the gratings become thinner and are not discernable to the infant.

In adults, the grating system has importance as it is used to determine the contrast sensitivity levels and also the hyper-acuity.

Method: The test is to force the infant or child to look at a 'pattern of high contrast'. When two dissimilar stimuli, one pattern and other blank, are presented, the subject 'prefers' to look at the pattern stimuli rather than a plain background. Based on the Teller's principle that the infant's vision is most sensitive to 'striped pattern', the cards are constructed having alternating black and white stripes, of increasing spatial frequency (varying width). The test consists of one card having the stripes and the other of homogeneous light grey colour, presented simultaneously from 1 meter distance in a normally illuminated room. A large screen has two cuts conforming to the size of the cards presented; and the observer looks through a peephole in the middle. The movement of the child's eye or head is noticed. The cards are presented for 5 seconds, and then another set is presented. In practice, if such elaborate arrangement is not possible, the cards can be shown simul-taneously, from 1 meter distance, and the movement of eyes or head noticed. Also now available, a large board which has one part striped and the other part blank, can be shown to the child (Fig. 5.6). To make the test more sensitive, the room can be darkened, and light flashed on both boards. But this is seldom necessary as the test gives fairly reliable results in normal illumination itself. The cards are commercially available, usually set of 8 cards (Fig. 5.7).

The cards have stripes of different widths, black and white, alternating with each other, and of diminishing widths. The last set of cards, having the thinnest stripes, which elicits 'no response' is the endpoint of the test. In other words, the last set of cards which the child can 'detect' and elicit the response, is the measure of the visual acuity.

Infants and small children are very sensitive to pattern stimuli and strongly respond to these patterns. Even if the head turns to one side during testing, the eyes move quickly in the

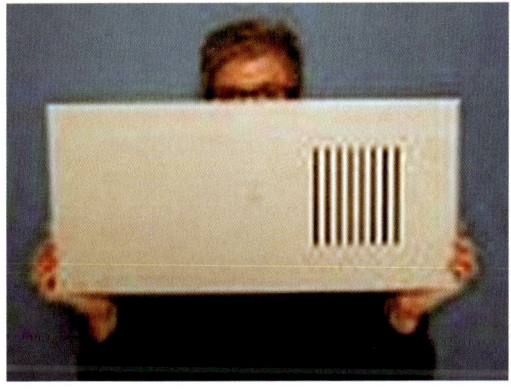

Fig. 5.6: Teller acuity card

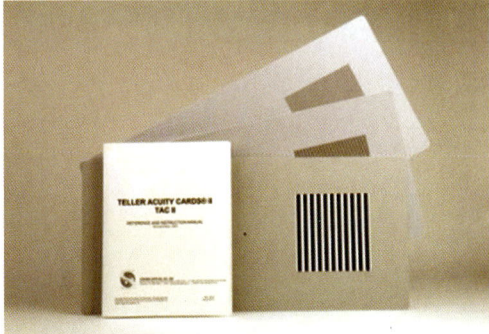

Fig. 5.7: Teller acuity card book

direction of the pattern card. It is noteworthy that how intently a child 'stares' at the pattern card.

The pattern of black and white stripes is also called 'square wave gratings'. It defines the limit of 'spatial resolution' capacity of the visual system in space. The name square wave grating stems from the transition between black and white are abrupt or 'square'. As already stated, the measure or quantification of this acuity is done as 'cycles/degree', as one black and one white stripe alternates at regular intervals or is 'cyclic'. As the width of each stripe decreases by a fixed amount (usually one-half), the number of stripes increase on the card. The finest or thinnest set of stripes that invokes the response is the measure of visual acuity.

The grating acuity also depends on the distance it is viewed, the light intensity in the room, and eccentricity in viewing.

In best standardized conditions, visual acuity of infant or a small child can be fairly well documented.

Figure 5.8 shows another variant of the concept of 'grating acuity' evaluation. The gratings can be inscribed on a ring type of thing, shown to the infant and reaction noted.

Cardiff Acuity Test

The Cardiff acuity cards, so-called because they were designed at the Cardiff University, byDr J Margret Woodhouse. It consists of a series of simple picture outlines, used to measure resolution

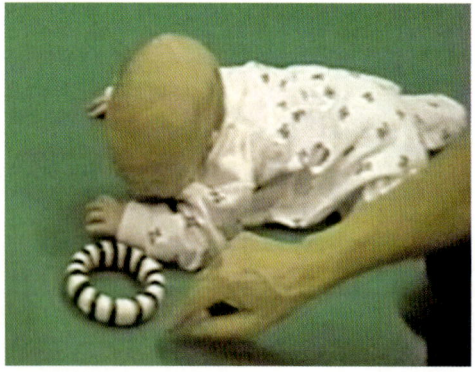

Fig. 5.8: Ring having black and white stripes for detection acuity in infnats

acuity in toddlers, and also in older children with mental impairment. The test is based on the same principle of 'preferential looking' and on the premise that a child when presented simultaneously with two different stimuli, will fixate on the picture pattern rather than a plain stimuli. The test uses pictures that will interest and attract a child. The pictures are so selected that they are familiar to the child which he/she sees daily, like fish, house, car, duck, boat, etc.

The Cardiff Acuity test consists of 3-set of 11 grey cards with six of more different pictures familiar to the toddlers, positioned at the top or bottom of the card (Fig. 5.9). Each picture's outline is a white band bordered by a black line and the mean luminance of these bands matches the card's background.

Each acuity level contains 3 cards with the same picture positioned at the top or bottom of the card. The set of cards are

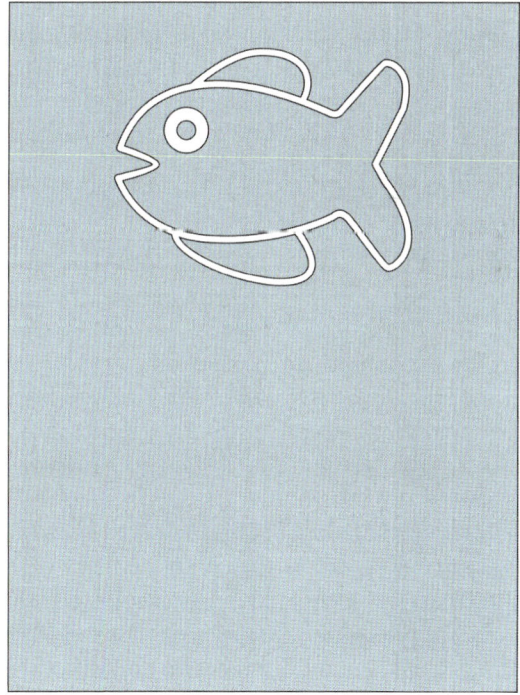

Fig. 5.9: Prototype of cardiff acuity card

labelled from A to K. To begin with, the largest picture set of card 'A' is shown. Three cards of the same set (same size) are shown to confirm the result. With correct response to the A card set, next 'B' set of cards are shown. This continues till no response to the pictures is observed. The picture set corresponds to the size of Snellen optotypes, with set A equivalent to 6/60 and K set equivalent to 6/6 vision.

The card is presented at child's eye level and the examiner watches the movement of the eyes. The card should be presented quickly and the abrupt eye movement observed. The picture can be sideways or up or down. The pictures become smaller with each successive card and the movement of eye is watched. The exercise may be repeated to confirm the previous findings. The specificity of Cardiff picture test is that it measures resolution plus detection acuity. Also the up and down place-ment of picture is helpful in estimating acuity in children with horizontal nystagmus.

Cardiff acuity cards are also used to assess the contrast sensitivity. Instead of changing the picture size, as in acuity testing, the white bands of the picture diminishes in colour from white to grey shades. The last picture, which cannot be visualized, gives the end point result.

Boeck's Candy Test

As the child begins to crawl, (around 1½ years) or begins to walk (around 2 years), this test comes extremely handy. Small pellets of candy, of different colours, are strewn on the floor and the child is asked to pick-up a specific one as indicated by the physician. Since colour vision is well developed after 6–8 months of age, a child whose vision is normal should be able to pick-up the specific candy. The test is quite reliable and gives a rough assessment of the acuity of vision. The test is more a qualitative analysis of vision, but it can be made of quantitative value by changing the size of the candy.

The author uses this test in a slightly modified way. Instead of number of candy's strewn on the floor, a 'single' small candy is placed on a white sheet on the ground; and the child is coaxed to retrieve the candy. The candy is the size of the 'gem' candy,

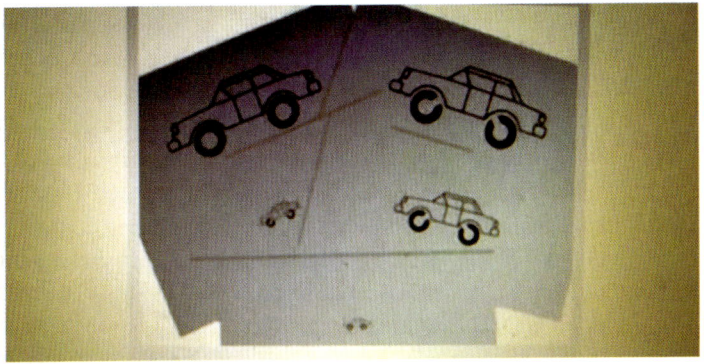

Fig. 5.10: Broken wheel test for acuity test in toddlers

and the child is observed as he/she goes to pick the candy. Different colour candies can be used and a child of 2–3 years should be able to pick-up the gem candy quickly.

The Broken Wheel Test (Fig. 5.10)

This is another test quite often used in 2–3 years age group, as the child now is quite conversant with motor cars and begins to understand its various parts. The child is simply asked to point at the broken point of the wheel of the car. On similar grounds, we have the Landolt's broken ring test which is used in vision evaluation of slightly older children.

VISION ASSESSMENT IN PREVERBAL GROUP

Lea Symbols

Introduction

Dr Lea Hyvarinen, a paediatric ophthalmologist from Finland, worked as a fellow under Dr Maumenee at Johns Hopkins Hospital, USA. She returned to Finland and became incharge of first 'Vison Rehabilitation Centre' in Helsinki, Finland. She now works as an Honorary Professor in Rehabilitation Sciences at the University of Dortmund, in Germany. She worked extensively to develop certain relevant tests for small children in the preverbal age group. She developed the Lea vision test system with specific Lea symbols for assessment of visual acuity in children. Later the Lea 'number' test was also introduced and now, the Lea test system contains an array of tests for different clinical test situations for children with multiple disabilities.

Among the many picture tests that exist, **Lea symbols** are the only tests that have been calibrated against the Landolt's 'C' vision tests. The Landolt's test is a universally accepted standardized optotype test used all over the world. It is identical to the 'C' used in the traditional Snellen chart.

The unique design of the Lea symbols and the special optotypes allow paediatric vision examination at a much younger age.

The Lea vision tests system currently contains over 40 different tests which target assessment of many different aspects of vision and communication deficiencies in children and adults.

The oldest and most basic form of test is labelled as 'Lea symbol test'.

The Lea symbol test: The test consists basically of four optotypes (test symbols) like the outline of an apple; a pentagon; a square; and a circle. Since these symbols represent an 'apple', a 'house', a 'window', and a 'ring'; they can be recognized at a much earlier age as the child is quite familiar with these objects (Fig. 5.11).

Lea numbers: The number test was the second in line developed to test the visual acuity of slightly older children, these conform to the principles of the Snellen optotypes.

Lea gratings: This is used to assess the 'grating or resolution' acuity and is helpful in children with severe visual defects or multiple defects. This is perhaps the only standardized test in brain damaged children that can reveal their limited capacity of processing number of parallel lines of high contrast only.

Lea contrast sensitivity: Visual information processing in low contrast levels is important to children for visual communication and understanding facial expressions in dim illumination as well.

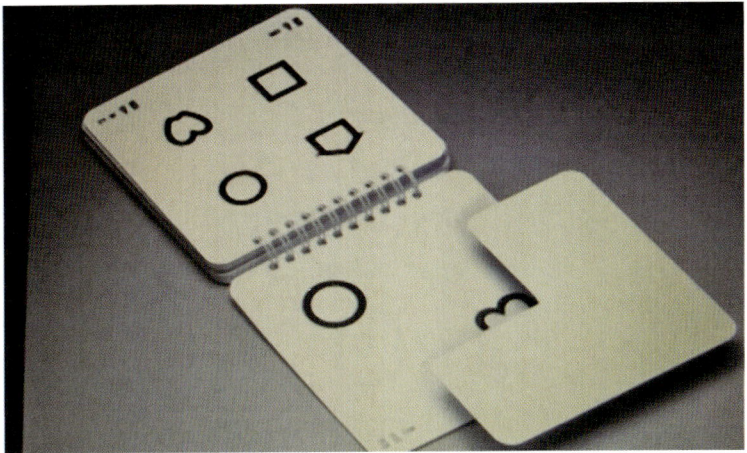

Fig. 5.11: Lea symbols

This test is a version of 'Hiding Heidi contrast face pictures' and depicts cartoon faces at different contrast levels.

Kay Pictures

Introduction

This vision test was developed by an Orthoptist, Hazel Kay, in the 1980s and has become the leading choice for vision screening and measuring preschool children's eyesight in UK and perhaps worldwide.

In 1981, when Kay pictures (Fig. 5.12) were introduced, the test was regarded as inaccurate and to be used only as a guide for vision testing in children. Then, over a short period of 2 years, more than 60 pictures were drawn according to the physiological principles employed in the Snellen charts construction, i.e. the component parts subtend 1 minute angle at the fovea, and the whole object subtends an angle of 5 minutes of arc. The more complex pictures required a 10 by 10 grid. However, quite a few pictures are now discarded owing to their complexity. The tests are reasonably accurate from 20 months to 36 months of age. Also Kay picture test now contains only those pictures proven to be both recognizable and accurate.

Children V.A. Test Chart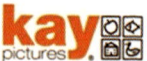

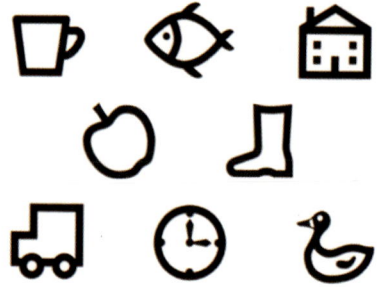

Fig. 5.12: Kay picture acuity test for preschool children

The Test

The 'Kay picture test' is a visual acuity testing system for children and adults with learning difficulties. The picture optotypes are proven to conform accurately with Snellen optotype design, for distance as well as near.

There are six comprehensive near and distance vision testing sets in the Kay picture range. Each set offers varying test distances, single or 'crowded' presentations and picture choice or notation.

The pictures are also available in a 'screening book' form having eight pictures, which the children could readily match with single picture showed to them.

A 'Crowded LogMAR test' is also available to test small degrees of amblyopia which can be missed by single letter test. It is presumed that by 3 years of age most children have the necessary concentration to achieve reliable results with the 'crowded picture test'.

The STYCAR Tests

Introduction

One of the most popular tests used for small children (toddlers) and adults in certain situations are the STYCAR tests, designed by Dr Peter Ambrose Gardiner and Dr Mary Dorothy Sheriden.

STYCAR is an acronym meaning 'Screening Test for Young Children and Retards'.

Dr Peter Ambrose Gardiner specialized in Ophthalmology from Guy's Hospital, London. His research on myopia in 1960s is well recognized. He worked as Ophthalmic Surgeon in Barnet General Hospital and as Research Fellow at Guy's Hospital where he evolved the 'Guy's Color Vision Test.' He then worked at the Moorfield Eye Hospital, where he dedicated most of time for caring of the disabled children. He co-founded the Eye Group of the Spastics Society with Mary Sheriden. He will be remembered along with Dr Sheriden for the universally used Sheriden-Gardiner vision tests for children.

Dr Mary Dorothy Sheriden, was born in 1899 and was the eldest daughter of an Irish General Practitioner. From an early age, she displayed interest in Medicine and finished her medical graduation from Liverpool Medical School. She began her career in a humble way as a medical officer in Manchester, England. She got disturbed particularly at the plight of hearing, speech and visually handicapped children.

Her expertise in the field of developmental paediatrics is well recognized. She developed the STYCAR tests, which in the modified form, are widely used to even today. Though being a paediatrician by profession, her extensive work for visually handicapped enabled her to win many laurels and awards.

She continued her research till her death in 1978.

The Test

For many years Dr Sheriden and Dr Gardiner tested several hundred normal and handicapped children with the currently available vision tests like Illiterate 'E' charts, Sjögren's hand and Landolt's broken ring charts, etc, only to discover that all had some pitfalls and severe shortcomings for large scale vision testing. Thus it became necessary to design new vision charts which could serve valuable purpose for both young normal children and handicapped children. The series of vision charts which were developed from these beginnings was given the name 'STYCAR'—meaning 'Screening Tests for Young Children and Retards'.

The original STYCAR test was composed of nine standard Snellen letters without serif, i.e. letters conforming to a circle, square or triangle. The letters thus selected (H, L, C, T, O, X, A, V, U); in accordance to the well-established psychological findings that a child is normally able to copy a vertical line at age of 2 years; a horizontal line at 2½ years; a circle at 3 years; a cross at 4 years; a square at 5 years; and a triangle at 5½ years. On the wall-charts, the letters are spaced well apart, with not more than 3 letters in a line. The letters measure from 6/60 to 6/6 and the charts are intended for testing at 6 metres. These charts worked well for children around 4–5 years of age but problems arose in testing below this age and in mentally handicapped children. The following 3 findings emerged:

a. Most of children found it difficult to maintain rapport for necessary time required for the test at a distance of 6 metres.

b. They responded more satisfactorily to a series of cards having only one letter (5" by 5") grid rather than the whole line.

c. Many children could not name or copy the letters but readily matched with a card shown to them.

Thus, the modified, currently used test includes 'single' letter card in 5" by 5" (5 min by 5 min.) grid shown from a distance of 3 metres and then the child is urged to match the letter from the cards made available to him. To further facilitate the process, fewer letters are shown from 3 meters. Also instead of letters, toys of different sizes or set of 10 graded balls are shown. The procedure is similar of matching.

With further knowledge regarding the response of younger children of preverbal group, and refinements made on selection of letters by other researchers like Dr Lippermann, the number of letters were reduced to four only and those letters were selected to which the children gave the 'best response'. Thus the letters selected were H, O, T, V, and the test came to be known as 'HOTV' test (Fig. 5.13) and is very popular in most of the clinics worldwide.

Landolt's Broken Ring Test

This test was developed by a Swiss born ophthalmologist, Dr Edmund Landolt.

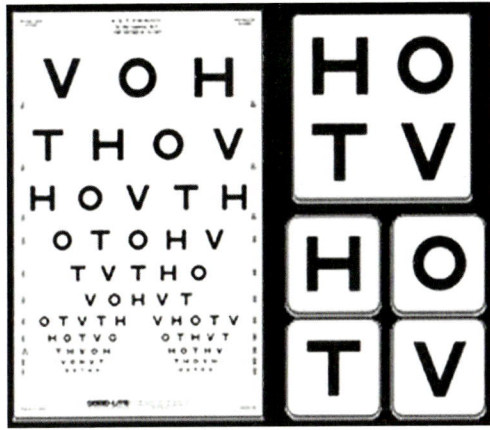

Fig. 5.13: Shriden-Gardiner acuity test for preschool children

The test uses the Snellen optotype 'C' as the standard test symbol. The only difference is that the 'break' in the ring is of the same width as the width of the limbs of C. Hence, it appears to be more similar to a ring rather than letter C. The placing of the break varies with each optotype or can be varied by rotating the optotype also, and the observer has to point at the direction of the break (Fig. 5.14).

Since the test utilizes a single letter which remains perfectly standardized in each line, it is supposed to be more accurate and is widely used as a standard test for acuity determination.

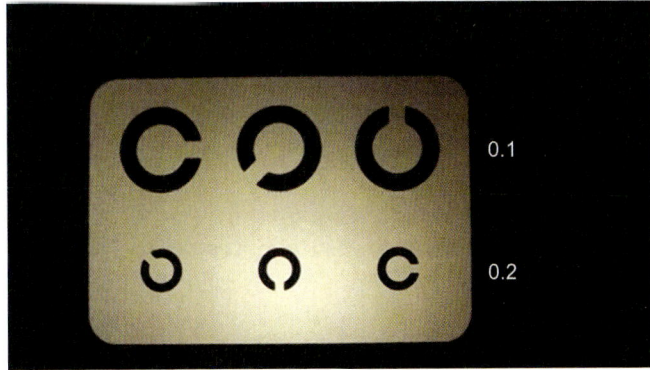

Fig. 5.14: Landolt broken ring vision test

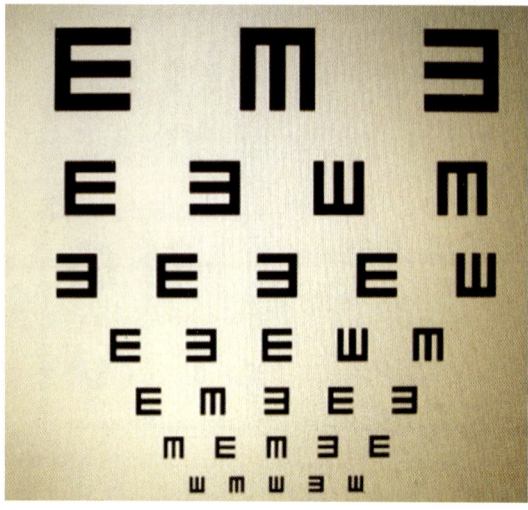

Fig. 5.15: Illitrate E-chart for vision testing

E-Chart Test (Fig. 5.15)

On similar lines as the Landolt's C chart, the letter 'E' of Snellen optotype is used for visual acuity assessment in the preverbal group. It can also be used in illiterate adults. The advantage of this chart, as in Landolt's test, the direction of the limbs of E can be changed, and, therefore, it is cheat-free.

Allens Figures

One of the most popular and extensively used test charts for a preverbal child are the Allen's figures (Fig. 5.16).

These are figures of different types which a child is seeing in everyday life and is well conversant of these objects. They all conform to the Snellen optotype size, and visual acuity from 6/60 to 6/6 can be quite accurately assessed. The chart is available for near testing also, again based on the Snellen principles of sizes at different distances. Object sizes corroborating with sizes for 3 meter distance viewing, are also available and routinely used, if it is found that the child is not able to maintain attention at 6 meters. Picture cards are available for viewing from near.

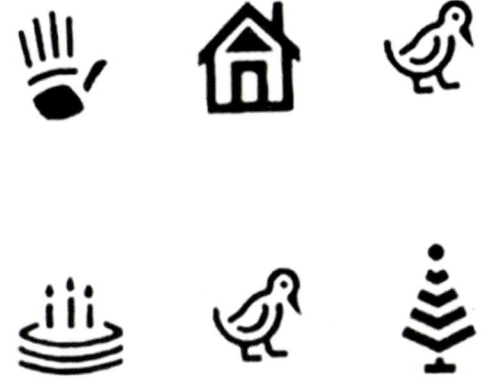

Fig. 5.16: Allen's figures

Various other clinicians came forward to device different types of charts depicting different objects, keeping in mind of child's preference to different objects he/she views around. An example is the Kentucky vision chart (Fig. 5.17).

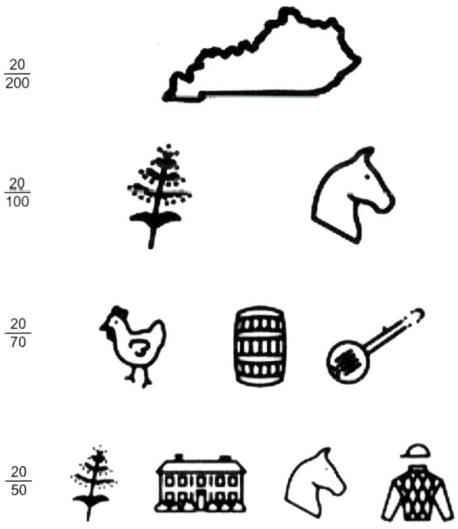

Fig. 5.17: Kentucky children's eye chart

ASSESSMENT OF VISION IN A VERBAL CHILD

Introduction

Around five years of age, 'recognition and resolution acuity' has reached the adult stature and child has well developed visual pathways and cognitive faculties, and is now able to identify objects and begins to read and write; and thus makes the visual assessment much easier. Based on this assumption, a number of charts have been developed, where a child can read letters, or numbers in line formation.

'Resolution' acuity is usually expressed as the smallest angular size at which subjects can discriminate the separation between critical elements of an object or a stimulus pattern such as a pair of dots or lines. Thus in a well-developed resolution acuity, a person can discriminate the finest limbs of any letter or pattern. For example, limbs of letter 'E' or 'N' can be identified to the finest order. The finer the parts of an object are identified, the higher is the visual acuity. As already previously mentioned, discrimination of more than 30 sec/arc or 40 cycle/degree is the now the function of the 'visual cortex' and is referred as 'hyperacuity'.

The most important person in the history of vision assessment is undoubtedly, **Dr Herman Snellen**, a Dutch Ophthalmologist, who, almost 150 years ago, devised a system of examining the visual acuity of a person, which has stood the test of time and is still considered the Gold Standard of vision assessment in children and adults alike. The different types of tests evolved over the years for testing visual acuity in children and adults, are all based on the basic principles of Snellen. It would, therefore be, not out of place, to give a befitting tribute to this great ophthalmologist of all times!

Dr Herman Snellen was born in 1834 in Zeist, Netherland and died in 1908 in Utrecht, Germany. Son of a well-known physician, he studied Medicine at Utrecht University under Dr Francis Donders and specialized in Ophthalmology.

Dr Snellen would ask people to gaze on charts on distant wall and would ask to report what they could see. It dawned upon him that people could identify objects of a particular size at specific distances only. He experimented with different sizes of objects and distances. For simplicity, he used circles, squares, etc., as objects in his testing charts. But people would easily interpret these and would cheat on these symbols. He then replaced these symbols by alphaneumeric letters. Painstain-kingly, he deduced that a certain letter of a certain size, when produced an angle of 5 min of arc on the eye, could be seen clearly at that distance. Also the elements or parts of a letter should be of certain width to be identified separately. And this width was found to be subtending an angle of 1 min of arc (of a circle). Thus the **Snellen Letter Chart** came into existence. The letters, known as optotypes, were calibrated and measured such that the smallest letter to be seen at a distance of 6 metres should be at least of 8.86 mm; and the smallest letter to be visible from 60 meters should be at least of 88.6 mm. Beyond 60 meters, the vision of a normal person was not appreciable, and hence that was supposed to be the longest distance for a normal vision. For less than 6 meters viewing, the letters could be made smaller but conforming to the standard 5 min of arc angle. The word 'optotype' signifies a standardized symbol used for visual acuity testing.

The Snellen Test Chart

Since the Snellen charts are most widely used the world over, it would be discussed in detail for better understanding. The distant vision chart of Snellen initially had 11 lines, each for a particular distance, and constructed in a 5 by 5 grid (subtending an angle of 5 min of arc). 'Arc' is part of a circle, conforming to the clock which has 60 minutes and each arc is of 5 minutes, which again has 5 parts in 1 min interval. Thus the whole letter fits into a 5 by 5 min grid and limbs of the letter subtending a visual angle of 1 min. Also the spaces between the limbs of the letter are of the same width, subtending the same angle of 1 min of arc. As we go down the lines, the size of the letters would correspondingly decrease but maintaining the same visual angle.

The thickness of black lines of letters equals the thickness of white spaces between them. The chart uses high contrast principle—white background with black letters, so that the contrast is 100%. Only ten Sloan letters are now used, viz. C, D, E, F, L, N, O, P, T, Z; presumably because they are more easily legible and which are better constructed of more uniformity. The sorrounding luminance is usually photoptic.

The test is conducted at a distance of 6 meters, and this figure is the numerator of the 'Snellen fraction'.

The denominator gives the distance in meters at which the details of letters in that particular line are readable. For example, the width of limbs and spaces of the letter 'E', on the designated line of 6/18, is such that they subtend an angle of 1 min of arc at 18 metres.

Standardisation of Snellen Chart

The Snellen chart has been criticised on number of grounds. Some letters are easily recognized than others; some are confusing like H and N. Each line has variable number of letters where by authentication of vision cannot be done. Some letters do not exactly conform to the 5 by 5 grid. Another uncontrolled variable known to influence visual acuity is the luminence, which has not been defined. Taking cognizance these short-comings, the Snellen charts have undergone modifications.

It is desirable to standardize the conditions under which the visual acuity testing is measured:

a. The variation in letters has been solved by using only a single letter 'E' in Snellen chart. This letter diminishes in size as we go down the chart. To some extent, this problem has also been solved using the ETDRS chart where each line has only 5 letters.

b. The controversy of letter size is solved by using the **Sloan Letters**, which are without serifs. Each line has the letters spaced equally apart and the spaces between lines is also equal. This has given uniformity in repeated testing of visual acuity.

LogMar chart: To further authenticate the testing of vision, more so the number of letters read in each line, the LogMAR system is now used in most of research-oriented testing. This system has already been dealt in beginning of this chapter.

The ETDRS uses Sloan letters with the LogMar system to further add specificity and fine tuning of visual acuity.

c. **'Illumination'** is one of the critical factors in determining the visual acuity. A Snellen chart should be amply illuminated in accordance with the norms subscribed. In most cases, the parameters are not adhered to. Modern day charts are usually self-illuminated or the projector is used, where the chart is projected onto a screen. Whichever appliance is used, it is important that the lighted chart or screen is in accordance to the standard norms. For the knowledge of the reader, a simple information is justified.

'Luminous Flux', measured in Lumens, is the total amount of light present or emitted; and 'Luminance' represented as 'lux', is the measure illuminating a given surface from a standard fixed distance. A flux of 1000 lumens, concentrated into an area of 1 square metre from 1 metre distance, lights up that square area with a luminance 1000 lux. However, the same flux spread over an area of 10 sq. metre, will provide luminance of 100 lux.

A standard Snellen chart should have luminance of 500 lux. Tests have been performed from luminance ranging from 50 to 500 lux and it has been observed that there arises a difference of 2 lines where illumination goes down to 50 lux. For practical purposes, luminance of anywhere between 400 to 600 lux is ideal for testing.

CONCLUSION

We have come a long way since Snellen, 150 years ago, first experimented to develop a system for recording of visual acuity. In the intervening years, numerous clinicians and researchers have developed their own charts for evaluation of vision in children, illiterate persons, adults, and handicapped persons. Various modifications have been done in the Snellen chart system also; but the basic scientific principles of Snellen for vision evaluation have remained intact. Whatever newer and more specific charts have evolved, are all based on the same principles of Snellen chart.

Though we now know that vision is not only 'visual acuity', and visual acuity is also not only 6/6, all acuity testing revolves round the 'angle which the object subtends at the fovea'; a concept first given to us by Dr Snellen.

Many different charts have been developed specially for small children; each researcher trying to device a way which are best suited for reliable results of visual acuity in different age group of children; but we are still far from what we can believe is the 100% visual acuity test. This is not easy, as small children and particularly handicapped children respond differently at each time of testing. Also there are numerable variables which influence the vision evaluation. Nevertheless, we have quite a good number of tests for evaluation of vision in infants and children; the important ones have been enumerated and discussed in this chapter; there are still more, but either they are replicas of the standard tests or have not been found very reliable, hence have been omitted.

Management of Refractive Errors

Early in life, the two eyes of infants normally grow in a highly coordinated manner towards an ideal refractive state, a process called 'emmetropization'. Evidence from many different species indicates that emmetropization is an 'active' process that is regulated by visual feedback by the eye's effective refractive state. For example, making the eyes of young animals artificially myopic with positive lenses or hyperopic with negative lenses, produces compensating ocular growth, that can within certain operational limits, eliminates the imposed refractive error.

The refractive state of the eye is dependent on the relationship between the axial length and the combined refractive power of the cornea and the lens. Axial length changes from 17 mm at birth to 23.8 mm in adult. To compensate for this increase in axial length, the cornea and lens flatten, so that the mean refractive power of cornea and lens decreases from 51.0 diopters and 35.0 diopters in the newborn, to adult values of 44.0 diopters and 18.0 diopters, respectively. With such remarkable changes occurring in these parameters, it is gratifying that the refractive state of the eyes remains fairly stable.

Premature infants are recognized to be more myopic than full term infants; the reason described is due to the more convexity of lens. The mechanism responsible for this lenticular myopia is unclear.

At birth, a full term infant, on the other hand, is hyperopic. In one study, 75% normal infants were hyperopic (ranging from +1.0 to +10.0 diopters) and 25% were myopic (from −1.0 to

–12 diopters). These large variations are not clearly understood. Another group of studies indicate gradual increase in hyperopia up to 5 years of age; thereafter a myopic shift occurs towards emmetropization. Though there are wide variations in this shift, but if the axial length increases without a full compensatory changes in the lens or cornea, myopia ensues.

Changes in refractive errors vary widely from individual to individual making it impossible to predict the ultimate refractive error. It is generally believed that if myopia presents before 8 years of age, then the child is at a greater risk of progression to high myopia (greater than 5.0 diopters).

Astigmatism is more common in infancy than in general adult population. Against-the-rule astigmatism predominates and is present in more than 70% of infants. Corneal curvature is the major component of infantile astigmatism. Longitudinal studies have shown a dramatic decrease in astigmatism with age, with most pronounced changes occurring by 2 years of life. Most of this astigmatism disappears by 6 years of life. There is alteration in type of astigmatism also; with predominance of 'with-the-rule' axis. Infants with higher degrees of astigmatism may not revert to normalcy, specially if the axis is oblique.

Numerous research studies on ocular growth and refractive errors in many animal species including monkeys show similarities in the course of emmetropization. The fact that 'form deprivation' produces axial myopia in children, as it does in many species, reinforces the idea that visual experience regulates human ocular development and can play a significant role in the genesis of refractive errors.

ROLE OF PERIPHERAL VISION

Research conducted a decade back on the effect of 'peripheral vision' or 'off-vision', showed that peripheral form deprivation can produce axial myopia at the central fovea, even in the presence of potentially clear images in the central retina and that an intact fovea is not essential for the recovery from experimentally induced refractive errors. It was observed that peripheral retinal images can play a role in determining whether one has an abnormal refractive state and that degradation of peripheral image quality may contribute to the genesis of common refractive errors like juvenile onset myopia. Studies showing experimentally produced foveal ablations did not interfere with the recovery from induced refractive errors, suggests that periphery can contribute towards emmetropization, even in the absence of functional fovea.

There are several explanations as to how the peripheral image quality affects foveal refractive state:

- One is that the expansion of globe occurs all over, influenced by peripheral form degradation and that the foveal region becomes a part of it.
- Another possibility is that vision-dependent growth signals are pooled across large areas of the retina. The major part of signals originate from the larger peripheral area and have a dominant effect on the overall growth of the eye.

Regardless of the fact that peripheral vision can influence eye growth, it has important implications for the role of vision in the genesis of refractive errors in children. In particular, it emphasizes that the optical state at the fovea may not accurately reflect the overall balance of visual signals that influence eye growth. Instead, as several investigators have suggested, it seems likely that off-axis variations in refractive errors or image quality could determine refractive development. For example, it has been reported that individuals whose eyes are more hyperopic in the periphery, presumably because of the geometry of the eye or the shape of the posterior globe, are more prone to development of myopia at the fovea than individuals who manifest relative myopic state at the periphery. Given that experimentally imposed 'hyperopic defocus' promotes axial myopia in monkeys, it is reasonable to speculate that hyperopic defocus in the periphery, like form deprivation, promotes axial myopia in humans. This scenario may also explain, at least in part, why myopic individuals have more hyperopic off-axis refractive errors than do non-myopes. Moreover, the fact that peripheral refractive errors can be quite large and are not typically eliminated by optical corrections for the foveal vision, may explain why myopia frequently progresses over time even when the central refractive errors are corrected.

In any case, it seems likely that peripheral vision should be taken into account in efforts to determine the role that vision plays in the development of anomalous refractive errors.

It has also been suggested that peripheral image quality should be considered when designing treatment strategies for myopia and hyperopia. All previous optical regimens have focused on manipulating image quality at the fovea and have been largely ineffective. However, given the influence of the peripheral retina, correcting peripheral optical errors or imposing specific peripheral refractive errors, may be more effective in controlling eye growth. For example, it may be possible to slow the progression of myopia in children by prescribing lenses that correct central refractive error and at the same time increase the curvature of field of the image plane, thus correcting the peripheral hyperopia or creating myopic defocus in the periphery! Both clear vision and myopic defocus in the periphery are strong stimuli for reducing axial growth. Similarly, prescribing glasses that impose hyperopic defocus in the periphery could be effective in promoting axial elongation in short hyperopic eyes.

If the above hypothesis seems logical, then the whole system of refraction and prescribing spectacles has to be reviewed. How can this be achieved, needs to be investigated and looked into. Now it is becoming clear why undercorrection in a child with a pseudophakic lens, leads to myopization of the growing eye!

MYOPIA

Myopia has emerged from ancient Greek word *'muopia'* from *myein* meaning *'to shut'* and *'opos'* meaning *'eye'*. It is also commonly known as 'near or short sightedness' in layman jargon.

Myopia is the most common refractive error and so prevalent that it has attracted the maximum number of studies worldwide. A recent study by National Eye Institute, USA, showed incidence of myopia in general population has grown from 25 to 41.5% in the last 30 years.

Looking at the worldwide figures, a whopping 70–90% prevalence exists in some Asian countries, 30–40% in Europe and USA, and only 10–20% in Africa. Besides these figures, there exists another devastating form of myopia in its 'pathological' entity.

The increase in the incidence of myopia and the futile measures to prevent its progression have generated a deep interest into its factors of pathogenesis, prevention, and management.

Myopia is a childhood disease and its progression is so gradual and insidious, that the problem goes unnoticed until it is advanced. It is only when the child's vision has significantly deteriorated that treatment is sought. For the most part, blurring of vision is the only complaint, and that too clears when the person approaches the object. Asthenopic symptoms, which are so pronounced in other types of refractive errors, usually do not occur in myopia. Even if these symptoms occur, they are usually due to associated conditions like astigmatism, muscle imbalance, or anisometropia. Since myopia is so important a disorder to affect such a large population of children, a detail enquiry into the condition is logical.

Etiopathogenesis

The greatest challenge that faces the clinician and the researcher alike is the progression of myopia.

Decades of research and the jugglery of clinical trials have not given any results as how to control the progression of myopia. We will now discuss about some of the reasons and speculations with which myopia progression is implicated.

Heredity

Heredity is an unarguably the most significant factor in causation and progression of myopia.

Linkage studies have identified 18 genetic loci on 15 different chromosomes that are associated with myopia. That means no single gene(s) are responsible for the disease.

Nutrition

Like so many dietary deficiencies or dietary anomalies linked with certain diseases, myopia also finds a place in the list. Poor diet, especially low protein diet, has been implicated for progression of myopia.

Hyperinsulinaemia, insulin resistance, insulin-like growth factors, carbohydrate metabolism disturbances, etc. all have hypothetical attributions in myopia.

Myopia and Near Work

Studies evaluating the association of myopia with near work have produced inconsistent results with regard to impact of near work on the development and progression of myopia.

First of all, the amount of reading and writing or for that matter any near work, to have a significant impact on myopia, has not been quantified. The number of hours of reading per week, as a causal factor for myopia, is debatable.

Secondly, the type of near work is also not defined. Does only reading and writing has an impact or other types of vocational near work is a contributory factor? Some researchers have found extensive reading accounting for a significant increase in refractive error, but the correlation was extremely low.

One hypothesis for a potential cause of myopia development was 'hyperopic defocus' from poor accommodation or 'accommodative inefficiency'. This theory has been tested by the COMET (Correction of Myopia Evaluation Trial) study, and other groups. The result seemed to be modest in these trials. In a more recent study, 'accommodative lag' was evaluated before and after the onset of myopia in a group of young children. But no difference was found in accommodative lag before and one year after the onset of myopia. Though all these studies may not align with each other, but general consensus among number of authors is that there could be a correlation between accommodative factors and myopia progression. Another interesting inference deduced from some studies is that 9–10 hours near work can be compensated by 2–3 hours of outdoor activity, as regards the myopia progression.

The results could be translated in that it may not be the reading time that is relevant to the risk of eventual myopia, but the amount of distance activity in which a person is engaged. The greatest deterrent to myopia in the presence of hyperopic defocus or overuse of effective accommodation for near work was the use of a 'plano lens', along with equal hours of outdoor activity. This experiment indicates that distant clarity of vision is more effective cue than near defocus in human eyes to retard the progression of myopia in children. The risk of any 'go' signal may not be relevant, if there is sufficient 'stop' signal to counter it! Thus the 'amount of outdoor activity' may provide the 'stop' signal.

On similar basis, the use of 'over convergence', in causation and progression of myopia, has been under debate. The pressure on the globe of contracting muscles for long time may, in some part, increase myopia. But this has also not been scientifically proved.

Another area that has been looked into is the significance of 'blood flow to the eye'. It has been postulated that increased blood flow, i.e. better oxygenation and nutrition, has an inhibitory effect on excess ocular growth. Sports or outdoor activity does not increase ocular or choroidal blood flow and, therefore, that related effect on the growth of eye does not seem possible. On the contrary, high axial myopes are advised to avoid strenuous physical exercise.

Intelligence and Myopia

Certain confounding effects must also be considered, e.g. myopia has been associated with other characteristics such as high IQ and type A personality. Children involved in endurance sports and other outdoor activity are more cheerful and extro-vert; a personality trait not found in children confined to room!

Again correlation between more hours of study and intelligence has not been defined. Children studying for more hours may not necessarily be intelligent. In some studies, it has been observed that children who studied couple of hours a day, and involved a couple of hours in outdoor activities, had higher grades than children who only studied.

Outdoor Activity

Some authors have argued the relevance of outdoor 'sports' in myopia. They question the reliability of 'sports' rather than simple outdoor activity of any sort. The idea, as it is argued, is not necessary to engage in sports only, but any non-sport outdoor activity which does not need accommodation or near focus, can also be a deterrent in myopia progression. A fact to which everybody agrees is that children with no parental history of myopia have almost no chance of developing myopia, provided they balance their indoor near work with outdoor activities.

The evolution of eyes has been going on for millions of years. Human eye, as many authorities suggest, was not programmed for so much of near work! The environment to which the human eye was adapted over millions of years does not match our present environment. Its function was to view landscapes, mountains, and meadows! The stress of constant near work, compounded by the use of computers and other near gadgets has increased, as speculated, the load on our eyes and the prevalence of myopia.

Lopsided reading habits, artificial lighting, reversal of biological clock, etc. all have contributed to increase and progression of myopia.

There is clear evidence that lack of normal stimuli causes improper development of the eyeball. The 'normal stimuli' refers to the environment. Modern humans, who spend most of their time indoors in dimly lighted or artificially lighted rooms, are not giving their eyes the appropriate visual stimuli to counter the abnormal eye growth.

Certain races in Africa and Arctic regions who mostly lead a life of hunting and wandering outdoors, have the lowest rate of myopia!

Gender Variability

Controversy exists in the gender variance in the epidemiology of myopia. In models produced for evaluating myopia in boys and girls showed that near work was not significantly associated with myopia but the number of sports/outdoor hours was inversely proportional to the progression of myopia. This was shown in one study where girls were affected more by myopia than boys, probably because of the less hours of outdoor activities than boys. In any case, it needs a more large scale, long-term study to substantiate these findings.

Illumination

Time and again, the issue of illumination has always cropped up. Parents and medical fraternity also have advised children to study in good illumination or well-lighted rooms. Again this part has not been carefully investigated; how much light is optimum for near work to avoid so-called 'strain 'on the eyes, has not been evaluated. Does studying or working in dim light causes myopia? People working in candle or lantern lights over centuries has not shown increase in the incidence of myopia. Then, reading in dim light causes myopia, is a myth? Good illumination increases the 'depth of focus' and definitely improves near vision; but does it contributes as a deterrent of myopia?

In olden days, when children and people did study in dim illumination—which was not routine, nor was it for long hours! Most of the work was done in daylight and whatever close work done in dim illumination, was compensated by ample amount of outdoor activity also, and probably this worked as a deterrent to the progression of myopia. This hypothesis we have already discussed.

With all said and done, illumination per se, probably is not a frontrunner for causation of myopia—as all modern homes have sufficient lighting. The main issue is the number of hours we are giving to close work in artificial illumination.

Retinal Image Degradation

The work of Weisel (a Nobel laureate) and Raviola showed that degradation in the retinal image in animals, had a myopia generating effect. In humans, retinal image degradation might be associated with myopia development. We have already discussed at length the effect of peripheral image quality on the development of refractive errors and its importance is well taken. More importantly, the change in the central vision or foveal image quality has been long known to be associated with myopia. Corneal scarring, partial cataracts, ptosis, high astigmatism, and other image clarity affecting conditions may in young eyes, produce myopia. Therefore, prompt remedial efforts should be made to correct these conditions. This hypothesis further emphasizes that since undercorrecting myopia creates loss of image clarity, this practice should be abandoned.

Seasonal Variation in Myopia Progression

An interesting report in IOVS Journal in 2014 showed that myopia progression slows in summer months than other months of the year. This was attributed to children involved more in outdoor life in summer vacations. This study further potentiates the hypothesis of importance of outdoor activity in preventing the progression of myopia.

Biomechanical Changes

Normally, the axial length of the human eye increases from 17 mm at birth to 24 mm at around 12 years of age. From an initial hyperopia, the refraction gradually changes to emmetropia—a process of normalization. We have already discussed that a growth-control mechanism exists, which can accelerate or slow down the axial growth in response to defocusing of the retinal image during the formative years of the eye. It has been suggested that this mechanism works by regulating the scleral extensibility through complex changes in the synthesis and degradation of the extracellular matrix components.

The biomechanical properties of sclera are determined by the contents and organization of proteoglycans (glycosaminoglycans) and collagen. Collagen accounts for about 80% dry weight of sclera. It is known that plastic deformation of tissues is directly related to the proportion of small diameter fibrils. The 'diameter of collagen fibrils' in sclera of myopic eyes is reduced as compared to normal eyes, as well as the contents of collagen and glycosaminoglycans.

Experimental myopia in mammals is accompanied by a decrease in the scleral content of proteoglycans and collagen, with reverse changes taking place during recovery.

In mammalian models of high myopia, a thinning of posterior sclera, decreased content of collagen-related amino acids and small diameter collagen fibrils is found.

In myopic situation, the eye grows by 0.3 mm axially with one diopter myopia; 0.19 mm vertically; and 0.1 mm in width. Thus the elongation is disproportionally axial, causing an egg-like appearance of the eye.

Pharmacologic substances are being tested experimentally and clinically which can control the abnormal growth of the eye by strengthening the sclera and preventing its dispro-portionate growth.

Classification

Myopia can be classified. The classification is simple and based on cause or the clinical appearance.

1. *Axial:* The increase in the overall axial length of the eyeball attributes to myopia.
2. *Curvature:* The increase in the corneal curvature results in myopia.
3. *Index:* Myopia occurs due to an increase in the refractive index of the refracting elements of the eye, mainly the crystalline lens.

Clinically, myopia can also be classified as:
- Simple myopia
- Degenerative myopia
- Nocturnal myopia
- Induced myopia
- Quasi-myopia
- Pseudo-myopia

Simple or Progressive Myopia

This is perhaps the most prevalent of all types of myopia. Simple or progressive myopia, usually emerges at young age and continues to grow till the end of teen age. There may be a spurt of myopia progression usually at puberty and nearing adulthood. Rarely, myopia once set, may not progress. But as a rule, there is always a progression of myopia, albeit gradually in most cases. If myopia has appeared before 7 or 8 years of age, then in most likelihood, it is going to progress. Also myopia of minus 6.0 appearing at this age is an ominous sign, and may progress to pathological myopia eventually.

Every clinician faces a question from every myopic patient that in spite of religious and constant use of spectacles, his or her numbers keep on increasing. For almost half a century, theories and speculations on the causation and progression, have abounded the literature. More theories have incubated more controversies, such as: Does accommodation influence myopia; how much outdoor life should a young child need to counter myopia progression; what is the optimum use of eyes for near work; does any diet or drugs will help to control myopia; what spectacle correction is needed for myopia; is there any measure to stall the progression of myopia?

The answers are as mysterious as the questions! The reasons for the causation and progression of myopia have been well dealt and explained above. Let us now deal with the management of simple or progressive myopia.

Management

The high prevalence of myopia as a significant public health problem emphasizes the importance of finding solutions that slow or control myopia progression. The mainstay of treatment options of spectacles, contact lenses or for that matter refractive surgery, do not control the accompanying eye growth or retard the physiological changes associated with the abnormal eye growth. Newer therapies by pharmacological agents such as atropine or pirenzepine are now being explored for control of myopia.

The bulk of evidence from well-conducted studies shows that overall most therapies for myopia have small therapeutic benefits that last for relatively short period of time or have significant side effects. Some therapies may be effective in a small subset of patients, but their broad based benefit has not been proven.

Treatment that are currently available to control the progression of myopia include spectacle correction, contact lenses, orthokeratology, and pharmaceutical agents. Many studies on these modalities have methodological limitations, and their results should be interpreted with caution.

Surgical options like PRK and LASIK only restore the distant vision, but they do nothing to control myopia progression.

In order for the results to be seriously considered, the trials have to be standardized. For example, they should include the following features: A concurrent control group; random assignment of control and treatment group; masking of investigations; standardized means of measuring myopia; a large sample size; small loss of follow up; and long-term effect assessment.

Nevertheless, here is a resume of each therapy.

Pharmaceutical Agents

1. Atropine

Atropine molecule, a plant derivative, is a non-selective muscarinic receptor blocking agent. The blocking of receptors causes inactivity of acetylcholine at these receptors, and thus paralyses of the muscles in the eye. Atropine acts at the sphincter muscle in the pupil and ciliary muscles of the ciliary body and perhaps some action on the connective tissue of the choroid also. The paralysis of these muscles persists till the action of atropine wears off, which may take 10–15 days.

Since atropine has shown promise and is now extensively explored as an anti-myopia agent, it is logical that we go into some of its details.

Its topical use dates back to the medieval ages when Italian women used atropine to enlarge their pupils to attract men! In late 1700s, atropine gained notice for its effect on accommodation. But both pupillary dilatation and cycloplegia represent problematical side effects, without any therapeutic effect on myopia control.

The earliest use of atropine for myopia control was hypothesized by studies of Bedrossian in 1960s and 1970s. This application was based on the concept that myopia originates by excessive near work and presumed excessive accommodation. Serious doubts were raised regarding its actual scientific role in reducing myopia and its limitations on curvature myopia and pathological myopia. However, the main reason for disregard of this therapy was serious side effects and consequent loss of follow-ups due to drop-outs.

The first authentic work on myopia control by atropine was published by Gimbel in the Canadian Journal of Ophthalmology in 1973. The treatment regimens varied greatly and was not randomized.

Nevertheless, the studies did show changes in myopia but were also stressed that the anti-myopia effect may be limited in duration, say for first 3 years only.

Challenges in clinical trials of atropine: Despite the flaws in early clinical trials, the promise showed by the drug to offer therapeutic respite, encouraged many studies of atropine for myopia control. None the less, no truly definitive study has been offered, largely due to ocular effects particular to atropine. Even in well-controlled, randomized studies, the papillary dilatation by atropine makes a truly double-blind studies impossible. Further, the cycloplegic effect of atropine requires use of bifocals or multifocals to compensate for the accommodation loss and as stated earlier, these lenses have their own growth-limiting effects, which must be taken into account in any atropine drug treatment. This effect cannot be ruled out as explanations for their slowed myopia progression. Experimenting on use of placebo and using single-vision or multifocal lenses on these groups did not show any substantial difference.

Another important factor limiting the results is ensurance of compliance. In one of large studies in which full compliance was of 70%, subjects showed minimal (0.08 diopter) change in myopia as compared to 0.25 diopter change in partially compliant group. The potential reasons for noncompliance are the tell-tale side effects of atropine.

Despite the aforementioned challenges, many published studies show that atropine treatment combined with multifocal lenses have the propensity in controlling myopia. The Atropine Treatment of Myopia (ATOM) study led by Chua Weihan and his collegues from Singapore Eye Institute is considered one of the most reliable study reports. The treatment was monocular, thus obviating the use of multifocals and removing the discrepancy of effect of multifocals, and the study used higher concentration of atropine (1%). The study found decreased myopia progression with negligible increase in axial length over 2 years treatment period. By contrast, the untreated other eye grew in length of 0.38 mm over the same length of period. Curiously, the retardation of growth was more in first year of treatment but attenuated in the second year. And in the year following the cessation of treatment, i.e. in the 3rd year, the rate of myopia progression in the previously treated eye was double than the fellow eye, but progression rate was still lower than the untreated fellow eye. This rebound phenomenon was explained on the basis of drug-altered receptor sensitivity.

Studies using lower doses of atropine in 0.1% and even 0.05% have been provocative, but no long-term or large group data are available so far.

Another important question is the effectivity of atropine as related to age. We have limited insight whether there is an optimum age for atropine treatment. Specifically, is the efficacy of atropine dependent on age, given that children exhibit more myopia progression than adolescents. In one relevant study, atropine therapy was done on subjects by age, and it was found that atropine was most effective in 8–12 years group and then in 18–21 years group.

Yet another query is regarding the efficacy of atropine on the extent of myopia. In published reports, the best results are obtained in myopia ranging from –1.0 to –6.0 D. Another study included children with –6.0 to –12 D myopia. Though the use of 0.5% atropine did show slowing the progression of myopia, but the control group was not large enough to testify the results.

In any case, children of any age who show progression of myopia are worth trying the atropine therapy for control of progression. The question of concentration and dose is yet to be solved. Further, long-term, large group studies, specifying the age for best results, need to be undertaken. Also, as in amblyopia, the upper age limit where atropine therapy can be instituted needs to be defined.

More recently, studies with much lower doses have shown more promising results. It is now well established that atropine in dose of 0.01% is equally effective in controlling myopia. In such low doses, pupillary dilatation and cycloplegia are negligible, and, therefore, is very well tolerated.

The mechanism of action of such low dose atropine is controversial and not well understood. Human eyes have muscarinic receptors distributed throughout the eye including choroid, sclera and retina. Though atropine is a non-selective muscarinic blocking agent but surprisingly this low dose has very minimum effect on M1 muscarinic receptors in iris and ciliary body but effective on other muscarinic receptors in other parts of the eye. Its effect on receptors in sclera and retina, is speculated to control physiological changes associated with myopia in these tissues.

Atropine creates a generalised depression in retinal functions, as indicated by ERG , initiating release of dopamine from cellular stores, which may cancel out presumed retinal signals that augment the growth of eye.

2. Pirenzepine

Pirenzepine is a selective M1 muscarinic receptor blocking agent. Its use in management of myopia progression has been under investigation for almost a decade. It holds promise that it could supplant atropine as an antimyopia treatment, but with fewer side effects. Pirenzepine is reported to have reduced mydriatic and cycloplegic effects in humans. Thus it has merit over atropine which raises long-term safety concerns associated with excessive light reaching the lens and retina. A large multicentric study reported in Ophthalmology Journal in 2006 that use of 2% pirenzepine gel, given twice daily, reduced the progression of myopia by almost 30 to 50% as compared to the controls. The study was conducted for one year in children of ages between 6 and 12 years. The drug, as approved in USA, has 0.5% concentration. Even with 2% concentration, the gel has been found to have clinically acceptable safety profile. But, similar to atropine, some side effects of long-term use of these drugs discourage the clinician on adopting this type of therapy for long.

> *Points to note* _____
>
> The mechanism of action of atropine and pirenzepine has not been established, but it is assumed that it is independent of their action on accommodation; and that it may depend on its action on receptors in the retina or sclera.

3. Other Antimuscarinic Drugs

Two other known antimuscarinic drugs, used extensively in ophthalmic practice—tropicamide and scopolamine, have also been reported to slow down myopia progression. In a recent study of 136 treated and 164 control group, nightly adminis-tration of 1% tropicamide reduced myopia by approximately 50%. But the study was not randomized and and long-term follow-up is awaited.

This drug, though, holds promise as with only night instillation the pupillary dilation wears off by morning and the cycloplegic action is of short duration.

Scopolamine is similar to atropine in side effects and the long-term studies are lacking.

Other Miscellaneous Drugs

Intraocular pressure lowering drugs have also been clinically tested for control of myopia, motivated by the data, though equivocal, linking myopia with increased IOP. Beta-blockers have been studied most extensively. In a best designed study in this category of 159 myopic children, using timolol maleate, no evidence in regression of myopia was found in a 2-year period.

Epinephrine, also lowers IOP, and has been tried as an antimyopic agent. Though the results are inconsistent, but no serious long-term studies have been conducted so far.

3-Methylxanthine: Xanthines are a group of drugs used in the treatment of asthma and related disorders. It is a metabolite of theobromine and caffeine, used as stimulants and broncho-dilators.

Interestingly, methylxanthine has been found in the chemical analysis of many meteorites, which have fallen on earth as extra-terrestrial bodies, which proves that it is present in outer space as well.

7-Methylxanthine, an adenosine antagonist, has been found to be working against myopia. Its mechanism of action is reported to be on scleral ultrastucture and eye growth, as reported from studies on rabbits. In a clinical trial of 68 myopic children, reported in *J. Ocul. Biol., 2008*, were given 400 mg of 7-methylxanthine (7-MX) daily for 24 months. Axial eye growth was reduced in children treated for 24 months as compared to treated for 12 months. Myopia progression slowed down during the period of 7-MX treatment, but when the treatment was stopped, both myopia progression and axial growth continued with variable speed. The results indicated that 7-MX reduces eye elongation and myopia progression in childhood myopia. The treatment is safe and without side effects and can be continued for longer periods up to 20 years when myopia progression normally stops. While the oral therapy and minimum side effects have advantages, but the effect on myopia progression is very small.

These children were under study prior to the initiation of treatment and their myopia progression was followed up. But the retardation of axial growth continued only till the treatment was under way. After discontinuation of treatment, the axial growth resumed its progression.

Spectacles

The magic of treatment still lies with the spectacles. A child who does not see anything on the school board, is exuberantly delighted when his/her vision becomes clear and crisp on wearing simple glasses. Spectacle correction is the mainstay of management of myopia. But it is easier said than done! There are lot of queries which surround the prescription of spectacles. Let us examine some of them:

a. *When to prescribe glasses? Look at the example:* **Parents** bring their 4-year-old child to the clinic with a simple complaint that their ward has recently joined school and always prefers to sit among the front or middle rows; he faces slight difficulty from back rows. His distant vision examination showed mild deficiency of OD 6/12 and OS 6/9, respectively. Cycloplegic refraction shows simple myopia of 0.75 OD and 0.5 OS. Would specks be advised? The options are:

- Many clinicians would defer prescribing spectacles, and would prefer to follow every six months.
- Parents would object to spectacles for such small numbers and at such a tender age.
- Other clinicians would prefer spectacles at the first instance, with a notion that near work would further increase numbers.

    The author has the following perception: Firstly, a good cycloplegia is mandatory before refraction.

    It is well known that small amounts of hyperopia present as myopic symptoms (*see* later). Also if the child does not relax his accommodation, the retinoscopy/auto-refractor would show myopia.

    Secondly, the family history is very important. If either of the parent is grossly myopic, then rapid progression of myopia is imminent; and therefore, spectacles should be prescribed.

    Consensus is now gathering to give correction on detection of myopia, not to wait for myopia to progress and cause symptoms.

b. *What to prescribe:* There was a trend earlier to prescribe a 'little less' for myopia. The trend did not have a rational basis. But with the new concept now emerging to reduce accommodation, this concept may look logical. But it should also be remembered that there are strong doubts whether accommodation is really involved in progression of myopia. Until we cross the turbulent waters, it is prudent to give the full correction for myopia.

c. *Exotropia with myopia:* In exotropia with myopia, early glasses are strongly recommended, as minus lenses would stimulate accommodative-convergence to help straighten the eyes.

d. *In phorias:* If the patient has a phoria, the refractive status and type of phoria should be determined.

In case of exophoria, full correction should be given to facilitate accommodative convergence. In case of esophoria, which may be due to use of excessive fusional convergence (which is common in high myopes), care should be taken not to over prescribe minus lenses, which can increase the esodeviation.

A proper correction of myopia may reduce the esodeviation by removing the near reflex stimulus.

A common practice in children is to remove glasses for near, which should be discouraged.

With simple myopia of couple of diopters, they see much clearer than their normal counterparts; but they then have to bring the object too close, again inciting the near reflex and making eyes esotropic.

Unilateral myopia: Consider the following example: A child of 6 years is discovered with defective vision, OD, during a routine school examination. Child is referred to eye clinic, and examination showed the following:

Vision: OD—6/18; OS—6/6. Cycloplegic refraction showed: OD—1.0; OS—plano.

Since the child had no complaints and as a simple myopia, glasses were not prescribed. There was no family history of myopia. But the parents were advised to report every 6 months.

A year and a half later, he comes back, now having problem in vision. Refraction showed: OD—1.75 D; and OS—plano. The given points should be considered:

• Since early age, the child was a myope. Since anisometropia was very mild, and not detrimental to his sight, glasses were not prescribed. But the parents were advised to show again after six months. The myopia progressed unexpectedly and is now a matter of concern. Full correction of myopia should be given and parents advised not to be casual for follow-up visits.

- Such cases rapidly loose binocular fusion and become exotropic or present with asthenopic symptoms. Since we do not know the trend of myopia progression, it is always prudent to give spectacles early and strongly advise parents to consult at regular intervals.

Quasi-myopia: Progressive blurring of vision does not always mean that myopia is progressing. When a child who is wearing high minus lenses, is brought to the clinic with complaints of diminished vision, two important aspects should be looked for. Firstly, the position of the spectacles and secondly the 'pantoscopic tilt'of the specks. (Pantoscopic tilt is the angle of the spectacle frame from the vertical.) It is common for heavy spectacles to slide down the nose; this will change the effective power of the lenses, as the vertex distance increases, and will have reduced distance vision. Similarly, too much tilting of frame or wrongly mounted frame on the nose will change the effective power causing diminished vision.

Pseudo-myopia: Pseudo myopia is a condition when the patient complains of blurred vision at distance and the manifest refraction reveals minus lenses, but the factual position is different! The actual state is revealed only after a cycloplegic refraction which shows 'hyperopia'. One of the most prevalent notions is that cycloplegic refraction is not needed in cases of myopia. This is unfortunately misleading. Cycloplegic refraction is as important in myopia as in hyperopia. It should be taken a mental note that cycloplegic refraction should be done routinely in all cases of suspected refractive error, at least for the first time.

A simple example will make things clear: A young boy of 8 years comes with the complaint of blurred distance vision, OU. His distance vision recorded was: OU—6/18 Snellen; manifest refraction showed OU–0.75 D. Minus lenses were prescribed and the patient advised follow-up yearly, as a routine. Within a week, the boy was back with headaches and watering. A cycloplegic refraction was performed which revealed the real story. The refraction showed a hyperopic error of +2.0 D, OU. Thus cycloplegia alone unmasks the true error; what appeared to be a low grade myopia, was actually a 'pseudo-myopia', created by the excessive ciliary tone to overcome hyperopia, and the extra minus lenses prescribed, further accentuated the ciliary tone causing asthenopic symptoms!

Over correction in a myope: In this situation, a clinician will encounter innumerable times in his practice. Complaints of ocular asthenopia by a myope is unusual, but not rare. If a myopic child complains of eye strain, then immediately focus your attention on overcorrection. A minus overcorrection can provoke symptoms by producing excessive ciliary spasm due to over accommodative effort. The symptoms would increase on near work, as the patient has to accommodate more to compensate for the minus overcorrection.

If the current glasses show more minus lenses than manifest refraction, then overcorrection is present. If the manifest shows more minus than cycloplegic refraction, then ciliary spasm is present.

A symptomatic myope, who has been wearing over-correction for a long time, may have so much of ciliary spasm that it is not always possible to rectify easily. The overcorrection has to be weaned gradually in steps.

A very pertinent question will still haunt the reader, that why an overcorrection of just 1.0 or 1.5 D minus, triggers asthenopic symptoms; whereas a hyperopic child of + 4.0 or +5.0 of same age, remains asymptomatic. This is because a hyperope had this condition since birth and has well adapted to it (remember all hyperopes of this degree do not have tropias or amblyopia).

He has learned unconsciously, a comfortable balance between the accommodation required to see clearly and the vergence needed to maintain fusion. Actually, he uses fusional divergence to counter the excessive accommodative convergence. As the child grows older, the hyperopia gradually decreases and so his accommodative demand and the accompanying convergence.

But for a myope who has been abruptly over-corrected produces an accommodative convergence, to which, being a myope was not accustomed! To counter the over-convergence (created as a part of over accommodation), the patient tries to counter, in vain, by fusional divergence. The tug-a-war, subsequently, creates the asthenopic symptoms.

Night myopia: During nightfall or in dim light, our refractive state shifts towards nearsightedness. This night myopia has been known for almost two centuries, but it is only recently that it has gained importance. Though its cause has not been fully explained, but being a distinct clinical entity, it should be understood.

Three separate factors operate at night when the pupils dilate, viz. accommodation, spherical aberration and chromatic aberration. But for all practical purposes, it is the accommodative element which matters most. At night or in extremely dim illumination, there is loss of retinal image contrast. A low contrast of image is incapable of stimulating the accommodation to focus; so it simply drifts into a resting state. This resting state is not 'zero' accommodation, but an 'attempt to focus'. This results in myopic state. The typical symptoms are blurred image with surrounding 'halos'. The halos represent defocused retinal image.

Management deals with estimating the night myopia and then giving the appropriate lenses.

The easiest and simplest way of estimating the night myopia is to do a retinoscopy in a fully 'darkened' room at one metre distance with the persons minus correction in place. The extra minus lenses needed to neutralize the error present, gives the final correction. Children rarely need this correction, and is narrated here for academic interest. But an important aspect is that children should always be encouraged to study in good ambient light.

Contact Lenses

There has been a historical change in the quality and material used in contact lenses, since they first came into existence in 1950s. The transition has been from rigid PMMA, gas-permeable rigid, soft HEMA lenses and now to higher quality polymers of great comfort. There is a big inventory from which a person and doctor can pick and choose the right type of lens desired.

All contact lenses of routine use are meant to replace spectacles, but we will discuss some special types of contact lenses which along with their cosmetic purpose also serve to retard the progression of myopia.

The possibility that myopia progression can be controlled 'optically' has seen a recent upsurge in interest in this field, driven in part by demonstration in animal models that positive lenses can slow eye growth. Thus certain specific type of contact lenses are now available which presumably retard eye growth and myopia.

1. *Defocus or dual focus contact lenses:* Also known as 'defocus incorporated soft contact' (DISC) lens. These lenses are suggested to have myopia progression preventive effect due to creation of a peripheral increase in power, thus minimizing the effort of accommodation, which supposedly slows down the myopia progression. Also known as 'dual focus' soft lenses, these have significantly less power at the periphery compared to the centre, and it is thought that this 'peripheral defocus' may reduce the tendency for excessive lengthening of the eyeball.

   A recent (2014) 2-year randomized study on 221 children, aged between 8 and 13 years, was conducted in Hong Kong. Patients were randomly divided equally, wearing single vision lenses and dual focus (DISC) lenses. The study showed myopia progressed more slowly in 25% of DISC lenses group, accompanied by less axial elongation.

   More recently, Cooper Vision (USA) has released the MiSight lens, a soft multifocal contact lens, which has concentric rings in periphery for myopia correction for distance and a plus addition in centre to decrease accommodation.

2. *High oxygen content lenses:* Studies have shown that children using soft lenses of low oxygen content especially in very young patient are at risk of myopia progression (probably due to corneal changes, diminution in vision and defocused image).

For decades, myopia progression has been reported in low Dk/t hydrogel contact lens wearers and to a lesser degree patients wearing silicone hydrogel lenses. A number of studies done on this subject have not been able to precisely formulate any guidelines for contact lens wearers in myopia. A large scale, multicentric, broad-based study of age-matched, similar myopic refractive status has to be undertaken to authentically prove the quantum role of different lenses in myopia progression control.

Clearly, quantifying the role of factors such as lens wearing schedule (daily or extended), lens material, subject age, and refractive status will have to be taken into consideration to determine the importance of each in the changing refractive error of contact lens wearers.

Some studies comparing myopic progression among low Dk/t hydrogel lenses and silicone hydrogel lens wearers have shown that contact 'material' also affects myopic progression, although the relative contribution of physical properties versus physiological properties (corneal oxygen supply) effects are not fully understood. In a study that compared continuous (extended) wear of up to 30 days of high Dk/t lotrafilcon-A silicone hydrogel lenses versus daily wear low Dk hydrogel lenses, subjects wearing lotrafilcon hydrogel lenses had significantly less myopic progression than in those wearing low Dk hydrogel lenses, after controlling the baseline refractive error and age.

If a child has to wear a contact lens for myopia correction, a high water content with high Dk value comprising of a material with the above qualities should be used.

Orthokeratology

Orthokeratology or 'Ortho-k' is a technique of fitting of a specially designed gas-permeable contact lenses that reshapes cornea. The cornea is gently reshaped while the lenses are worn overnight, and the vision remains clear during the day after the lenses are removed in the morning. This, though, is a temporary effect; the vision remaining clear till the time the lenses are continued to be worn every night and reverts back once the lenses are discontinued.

The history of orthokeratology dates back to 1940s when scientists like Jessen, Nolan and Grant discovered that hard or PMMA contact lenses could reshape the cornea.

George Jessen was probably the first to produce a 'ortho-k' lens made of PMMA material which he marketed as 'orthofocus lens'. These early designs did not give predictable results partly because with PMMA material, the lens could not be worn for long hours and secondly the lens design made wearing uncomfortable.

However, it was not until computerized corneal topography became available in 1990s that it became possible to create designs with repeatable and effective results. Furthermore, the development of new base material for 'rigid' gas-permeable lenses with higher levels of oxygen permeability, opened up possibility of orthokeratology becoming an effective, dependable, and comfortable procedure. Finally, the introduction of computer-controlled precision lathe machines opened up avenues of not only high accuracy lenses, but also mass production and commercially viable lenses.

Throughout the last decade, a number of organizations related to orthokeratology are conducting research into the use of ortho-k lenses to slow down or prevent altogether the progression of myopia.

It is postulated that 6 micromillimetre flattening of corneal curvature results in 1 diopter of changed vision.

Therefore, a specially shaped lens can be used to lightly press on the cornea causing it to gradually flatten and configure it to a correct shape for a clear focused vision. This therapy is also known as 'corneal refractive therapy' (CRT).

Orthokeratology and CRT are theoretically different terms. CRT uses a specific brand of corneal reshaping lens (Paragon CRT), and has a proprietary lens design and fitting procedure. Though technically different from orthokeratology, the ultimate purpose is similar and produces comparable results.

Another technique employed in orthokeratology is to use gas-permeable rigid lenses with increasing base curves over a period of time. The principle is to gradually flatten the cornea with different lens designs which would gently press the cornea, over a period of time. On removing the lens, the result does not last for more than 72 hours.

Ortho-k lenses have been successfully used to correct various types of refractive errors and retard the progression of myopia.

Points to note

With all said and done, orthokeratology has not stood the test of time. Unpredictable results, no lasting effect, and limited use have put this technique on the back seat.

Refractive Surgery

Laser refractive surgery: As lifespan is increasing and people living longer, their zest for a quality life is also increasing. Thus, more and more people, past 50 years, are consulting for laser treatment to get rid of their glasses. As trite as it sounds, age is only a number. And if the eyes are otherwise healthy, there is no sound reason why that person cannot get rid of glasses, if wishes so!

At the other end of age spectrum, we have children; some of whom have significant refractive errors; which are hampering normal development of vision and creating psychological problems. Apart from the medical issue, younger and younger people are seeking cosmetic procedures—a trend spilling into ophthalmic practice also. Yet this is an area where an ophthalmologist has to trend cautiously. Majority of refractive surgeons agree that 18 years and above is a safe age for laser refractive surgery. Some surgeons prefer 21 years as the lower limit before they embark for LASIK; while others tread more cautiously, giving a 2-year period, after 21 years age, for refraction to stabilize before going for LASIK.

Nevertheless, there is a small subset of younger people, where LASIK may be indicated to save sight. These are children with high hyperopia; high anisometropia; and high myopias. In these cases, either glasses are not helpful or contact lenses were not tolerated.

To date, roughly 15 clinical case studies have been published that report results of refractive surgery in children. Most of them have been for severe anisometropic amblyopia, where contact lenses were contraindicated due to some surface pathology or due to intolerance. In cases of high hyperopia, undercorrection was done due to limitation of lasik correction in hyperopia. Some surgeons preferred surface ablation than cutting the corneas in laser surgery. But this resulted in corneal haze. There are no concrete guidelines on refractive surgery in children regarding the safe age and type of refractive surgery. Also there are not enough data to conclude how a paediatric cornea responds to refractive surgery and same conclusions cannot be drawn for safety and efficacy of refractive surgery in children as we can do for adults.

Intraocular Contact Lenses (ICL)

This is a great procedure which has turned out to be a good alternative to refractive surgery. The advantage is that the lens is removable, if need arises. In cases where ICL does not fully correct vision, LASIK can be done in addition to 'fine tune' the results. The material used is biocompatible, plastic polymer, used as in any soft foldable intraocular lens. The lens is placed in the posterior chamber of the eye, behind the iris, with haptics in the ciliary sulcus.

Pathological Myopia

Pathological or 'degenerative myopia' and 'progressive myopia' are two different entities, and a clear distinction exists between them. Progressive myopia may gradually progress to minus 8 or 10 diopters, yet is not associated with any degenerative changes in the eye. Pathological myopia, on the other hand, is high myopia with choroidal and retinal degenerative changes. Both have strong familial predispositions, but their genetic patterns are different.

There is no known concrete treatment for pathological myopia till date. All the measures employed for restricting the progress of myopia, even judiciously instituted, remain in vain. Surgical procedures like strapping or 'bolstering' the sclera with cadaveric scleral straps, have not yielded any positive result.

Medical conservative measures, like vitamin A, antioxidants, calcium or vitamin D, have yielded anecdotal results. At best, some optical adjustments can be done like 'undercorrecting' the myopia which enables the patient to achieve higher magnification by bringing the reading material closer.

In pathological myopia, the patient is usually visually handicapped and needs assistance with 'low vision aids'. The time when this need arises, is past the teen age, well into adulthood.

In children, pathological myopia should be suspected when there is a rapid increase in numbers, history of similar type of myopia in the family, and a distinctive appearance of the fundus. Usually, the fundus shows tessellations, large disc crescents, and a circular reflex at the posterior pole where ballooning begins to appear. B-scan also shows a growing posterior elongation of the globe. Peripheral retinal degenerative changes, endangering sight, usually appear in the 3rd decade of life; and the parents of these children should be cautioned about these developments.

HYPEROPIA (HYPERMETROPIA)

Hyperopia or hypermetropia as is usually called, though not as common as myopia, but still is a significant and perplexing eye problem. In myopia or astigmatism, the patient comes with a clear cut vision problem; but in hyperopia, the patients vision is mostly normal but complaints of ocular asthenopia are prominent. Many times, these are so vague that easily overlooked. This is exactly what is happening in a busy outpatients department. If you start refracting these patients with cycloplegia, you will be amazed to find that how many of these patients you were missing. Even after successfully detecting hyperopia in a young patient, who has no vision problem, a dilemma exists as to how and what prescription is to be given. You will be left confused, that after all your labour and efforts to detect hyperopia and judiciously prescribing spectacles, the patient comes running back that his vision with glasses, on the contrary, has become blurred! Thus, hyperopia management is not as simple as it appears and the management has to be individualized and carefully titrated.

Definition

In hyperopia, the optical power of the unaccommodating eye is weak to form a clear image of the distant object on the retina. But this is easily compensated in most cases by using the power of accommodation. This may not be possible in all cases; and the excessive accommodative effort exerted to overcome the deficit, causes a basketful of asthenopic symptoms. In a recap, let us go through some of the basic features of hyperopia. Some terms used in hyperopia, like total, latent, absolute, manifest and facultative, need to be understood. It will be simpler, if we describe them through an example: Suppose a teenage patient comes to the clinic with complaints of fatigue and headache. The unaided vision is 6/9 OU, and the manifest refraction is OU +4.0. A cycloplegic refraction is done, which now reveals +6.0 OU. The patient is called back for a post-cycloplegic test. Now, putting +1.0 on each eye in the trial frame, the vision improved to Snellen 6/6 each eye.

The explanation is as follows: The total refractive error discovered with cycloplegia is OU +6.0, and this is 'total hyperopia'.

His plain refraction had showed OU only +4.0, and this is the 'manifest' hyperopia; and the remaining, +2.0, which was revealed only after cycloplegia, is the 'latent' hyperopia. From the +4.0 manifest part, the person is compensating most of it, i.e. +3.0, by his faculty of accommodation and is called the 'facultative hyperopia'. What remains is the +1.0 D, which he needs as an outside help to bring his vision to normal, 6/6.

This part of hyperopia which cannot be overcome and corrected physiologically by accommodation is called the 'absolute' hyperopia.

Etiopathogenesis

Etiopathogenesis of hyperopia is a short story as compared to myopia. But its understanding is important from both the clinician and more so from the patient point of view.

Hyperopia, basically, is the defect in the manufacturing of our eyes—short, small eyes with sometimes flatter corneas. As age advances, the crystalline lens grows in size; the accommodative effort increases the lens curvature, and makes the anterior chamber and the angles more and more shallow and predisposes to an attack of glaucoma. This book is not supposed to venture into the domain of advanced age, and so let us examine what happens to an hyperopic young person.

Children are born hyperopes. We know that at birth the average size of an eye is 17.0 mm; it rapidly attains 20.0 mm by end of first year, and by three years attains almost the normal size of an adult eye, 23.0 mm. It further grows, albeit, very slowly by about 0.5 to 0.75 mm by 12 years of age.

The corresponding large hyperopia in children is easily overcome by more than adequate accommodation. It is only when the error is too big to overcome or the demand of accommodation is too large, the symptoms of hyperopia ensue.

So, let us examine the situations in which the child will need medical assistance:

a. Diminished vision, in one eye or both, noted accidentally in school examination or elsewhere.
b. Strabismus
c. Unexplained red eyes, watering, irritation, etc.
d. Headaches, especially after a days work, in the evenings or after school.
e. Nystagmus.

Since each of the categories has a different set of management, let us explore each of them.

a. *Diminished vision:* Whenever diminished vision is reported in a child below 5 years and a cycloplegic refraction shows high hyperopia (+5.0 or more), then appropriate specks, as per the child's subjective correction, are given. It is to remembered, as a word of caution, that in normal situations even hyperopias of this amount are easily compensated by accommodation. Thus the child should be further investigated as to why his accommodation is faltering. There are certain neurological diseases where the accommodation may be affected. Also many systemic medications given to a child for epilepsy, GIT disturbances, antidepressants, antipsychotics, etc., all affect the accommodation. A careful history and interrogation of a child taking treatment for any other ailment should be asked.

Whenever, anisometropia and amblyopia are detected, appropriate management should be instituted.

There is another group with high hyperopia, normal but intermittent diminution in vision, especially after long hours of study or in late evenings. These children need some help with glasses particularly during near work.

As mentioned in the Chapter 9 on Accommodative Anomalies, children and adolescents are not immune to accommodative insufficiency; and this point should be kept in mind when unexplained ocular symptoms ensue in a hyperope.

b. *Child with esotropia:* Anisotropic child requires cycloplegic refraction with atropine 1%, and full cycloplegic correction. It is mandatory to detect the full hyperopia. In spite of full cycloplegic correction, there might remain a small amount of esodeviation. It is not necessarily non-accommodative component of esotropia. These children have to undergo another cycloplegic refraction after 3 months of wearing specks, and surprisingly some 'more' amount of hyperopia is discovered. New prescription is given, and with all accommodative effort now eliminated, the child will become orthotropic.

There is a general tendency to correct 'little less' in cases of high degree of errors. This thought has generated because of sympathy towards a small child wearing such high numbers, parents pressure to reduce numbers or simply out of fear that the child may not tolerate such high numbers. These notions are contrary to proper treatment; and it is stressed that a child's adaptability is amazing and is remarkable how well a child tolerates such high numbers. Most of times, a child may himself demand for his/her glasses immediately on waking up.

Small subtle changes in the alignment of eyes, especially in cases of hypermetropia (producing accommodative esotropia), may be difficult to diagnose. One of the simple but reliable test is the 'Bruckner's reflex'. It is an altered reflex of the fundus glow which occurs in cases of refractive errors and/or mild strabismus. Eyes with refractive errors show more pronounced reflex in hyperopia and pale reflex in myopias. In strabismic eye, the reflex is more red than a normal eye. The test has to be done in totally dark surroundings with a normal pupil size (Fig. 6.1).

c. *Headache,* though not as common a symptom in a child, as in adults with hyperopia, but demands a thorough cycloplegic refraction, whenever a child complains. Usually such complaints emerge in the evenings when the child is doing homework, already fatigued by the day's work; or after coming home from school; or intermittently, whenever overload occurs on accommodation. In all above situations, an appropriate cycloplegic refraction should be done. If a

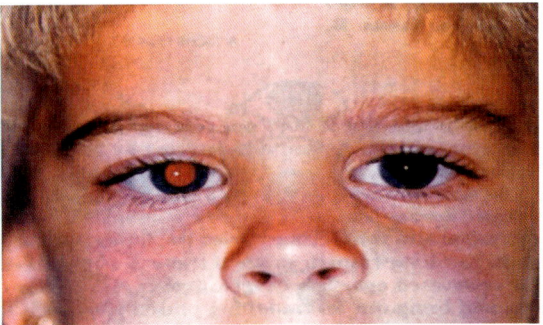

Fig. 6.1: Bruckner test

significant error is detected, then initially suitable specks should be given particularly for near work when the child is doing homework. Hyperopic glasses may not be needed full time, as they may hamper distant vision.

d. *Other ocular asthenopic* symptoms like redness, burning, irritation, itching, watering, etc. may accompany headaches or may occur independently. Exclusion of related ocular problems like allergies, infections, blepharitis, etc. must be carefully looked for and excluded. If still unexplained redness or watering continues, then a full cycloplegic refraction is warranted.

e. *Nystagmus,* though an unusual manifestation of hyperopia, but must be kept in mind when manifest and occult nystagmus is detected.

f. *Strabismus:* Almost 50% of hyperopic children present with strabismus, mostly esotropia.

These children may also have varying degrees of strabismic and/or anisometropic amblyopia.

In any case, both have to be treated, first amblyopia by occlusion and then esotropia (accommodative) by giving 'full cycloplegic correction'. In selected cases, where abnormal AC/A ratio is present, proper 'bifocals' have to be prescribed with certain regulations to be followed in spectacle manufacturing.

The hyperopic anisometropic child: A child may present with different magnitudes of refractive error in the two eyes. Let us examine two examples:

1. *First example:* A child of 5 years has the following findings: Vision—OD 6/6; OS 6/12 (uncorrected); *cycloplegic refraction*—OD +2.0D; OS +4.0D

There are two options:

a. To give full correction in both eyes. The child's RE has normal vision without any correction; now by giving unwanted plus numbers, the vision may become blurred in the RE.

b. Since the child has no complaints of asthenopia whatsoever, correction in RE eye is not needed. As a matter of fact, correction of only + 2.0 in LE will correct the vision, as there is a mild amblyopia in LE. This principle is generally adopted and stems from the rule that accommodation always works according to the better eye. For example, to see clearly at distance, OD accommodates by +2.0 D and 'simultaneously' OS also accommodates by +2.0 D. The remaining +2.0 D for OS to see clearly is compensated by specks.

2. *Second example:* A child of 5 years has the following findings: *Vision*—OD 6/9; OS 6/36; *cycloplegic refraction*—OD +2.5 D, OS +6.0 D.

   With correction: OD +2.5 D –6/6P; OS +6.0 – 6/24 only

The LE is showing moderate amblyopia. Here full correction of LE hyperopia is needed with initiation of amblyopia therapy. Since amblyopic eyes accommodate poorly, full correction of +6.0 D has to be given in LE. Gradually, as amblyopia improves and the vision comes to normal in LE, the prescription has to be titrated.

ASTIGMATISM

Astigmatism is perhaps the most misunderstood vision problem. Perhaps it is not 'a-stigmatism', but 'stigmatism', as there is some stigma attached to it! And, truely speaking, it creates the maximum problem amongst all types of refractive errors, as small amounts of error are difficult to detect on routine clinical evaluation and the symptoms are sometimes so vague, that they skip attention.

Etiopathogenesis

Basically, light fails to form a single focus on the retina to produce a clear image. Instead, multiple focal points occur, either in front or behind retina or on both sides. Thus the image formed is either blurred or distorted.

In majority of cases, it is the irregularity of the corneal curvature which produces defocused image. Sometimes the tilting of the crystalline lens or rarely its curvature can produce astigmatic effect. Very rarely, edema of the macula has been known to produce hyperopic astigmatism.

Usually, the aberration meridians in corneal curvature lie perpendicular to each other and is called 'regular' astigmatism. The steepest and flattest meridians are then called the 'principal axis'. If the axes are not perpendicular to each other, then the term 'oblique astigmatism' is used. In certain cases, multiple meridians from varying curvature exists, it is then termed as 'irregular' astigmatism. The uneven surface of cornea causes uneven refraction, leading to improper focusing. Such a surface is called a 'toric' surface.

Prevalence

In true sense, astigmatism in children is more prevalent than expected. In a study in USA on 2500 children, aged 5–15 years, 28% had astigmatism. In a study on a large population of 11,000 children wearing glasses, 47% had astigmatism of varying degrees in one eye and 24% had astigmatism in both eyes. In another study in USA taking ethnic population into consideration, Asian population had the highest percentage, followed by White race and then African race.

In a recent study done in India with rural base on 500 children aged 5 to 15 years, a whopping 58.6% were found to have astigmatism in one eye and 27% in both eyes. This corroborates well with other broad-based studies.

In a significant study conducted by NIH (National Institute of Health, USA) showed 24% had astigmatism in the age group up to 1 year, but only 10% had the error above 3 years. It, therefore, suggests that children outgrow their astigmatism with age.

Types of Astigmatism

When a single meridian or both meridians focus in front of retina, it is termed as 'simple or compound myopic astigmatism', respectively.

When one or both meridians focus behind the retina, it is termed as 'simple or compound hyperopic astigmatism' respectively.

When one principal meridian focuses in front of retina and other focuses behind the retina, then the term 'mixed astigmatism' is used.

'Irregular astigmatism'—perhaps the most annoying of all types of astigmatism, results when multiple focal points occur, either in front or behind the retina.

Clinical Features

The most common complaint in children is of headaches or eye aches. In fact, any of the features of 'ocular asthenopia' can manifest, like headaches, browaches, watering, red eyes, vertigo, irritability, sensitivity to light, drowsiness. Perhaps, complaint of vertigo and irritability after working or reading for sometime is the most distinguishing feature as compared to complaints with hyperopia. Visual complaints relate to the intensity of astigmatism. Small amounts of astigmatism may not manifest as diminished vision, but they all present asthenopic symptoms.

'Squinting ' is quite often reported by parents when the child is reading or watching TV. Squinting is NOT strabismus; it is narrowing of the palpebral aperture. It is an attempt to compensate or correct the corneal meridian in order to see clearly.

When any of the above symptoms are reported, a thorough cycloplegic refraction should be done.

Management

The following modes of treatment are available to correct astigmatism: (1) Glasses, (2) contact lenses, (3) LASIK and (4) corneal collagen crosslinking.

Glasses

We have learnt that astigmatism is more prevalent in infants and small children and gradually weans out or is reduced with age. Whenever spectacles are contemplated, the patient's acceptance is to be considered. There is always a dilemma that 'crisp' vision is more important than the 'alleviation of symptoms'. In a young child, where the question of amblyopia also comes into picture, good vision is preferred. Therefore, clinical experience and literature shows that 'full refractive' correction with glasses is always tried, so that the patient gets best vision possible. Children have remarkable ability to adjust to high refractive errors; and once this is achieved, their symptoms will also disappear.

Most of the astigmatism in children is 'against the rule', myopic or hyperopic.

Here is *an example:* A young girl of 7 years came to the clinic with complaints of headaches on watching T.V. She had spectacles prescribed a few months back, which exaggerated her symptoms.

Her present spectacles showed: OD–5.0/+3.0 140 axis– 6/9; OS–4.50/+3.0 140 axis–6/12.

Cycloplegic refraction showed: OD–3.0/+4.0 140; OS–3.0/+4.0 150

Two points are deduced from the previous prescription. First, the prescription is over-minused, which creates its own problems. Secondly, cycloplegic refraction shows its magic by showing us the correct path. With lowering the minus numbers and using the 'best subjective' correction technique, the problem was solved.

Example 2: A young boy complains of diplopia on reading. The present prescript shows: OD–2.0/–1.0 90 axis 6/6; OS –2.0/–4.0 90 axis, 6/6p.

On examining the glasses, they were too big, on a large frame. In this instance, the large frame produced 'prismatic effect' in the left eye on looking down on reading. This prismatic effect induces phoria and thus the headaches. The need here is not to reduce cylinders in left eye, as the vision is perfect; but to reduce the size of the frame. In high cylindrical prescriptions, this should always be kept in mind and clear instructions should be given to the optician not to give a large frame.

The following points should be noted during prescription of cylindrical lenses.

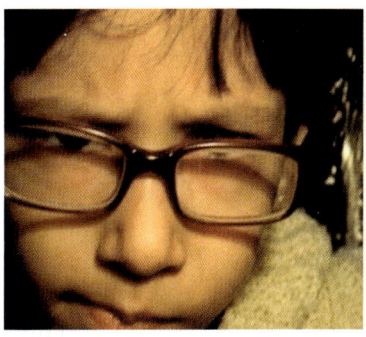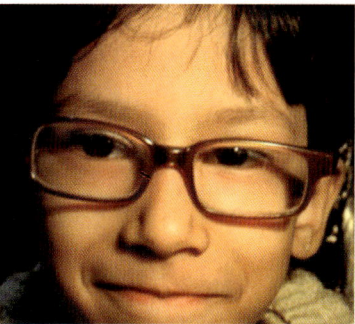

Fig. 6.2: Illustrations of spectacles—shows incorrect way and correct way of wearing specks. The effect is most pronounced in astigmatism.

a. *Lenses:* Size of the glasses should neither be too large nor too small. Large lenses create prismatic effect on movement of eyes in different directions.

b. *Frames:* The size of the frame should also be specified. Larger frames invite larger lenses with its own inherent problems. Large frames also have the tendency to tilting, which changes the axis of the cylinders, and causes asthenopic symptoms.

c. *Pantoscopic tilt:* Pantoscopic tilt is the line of plane of the frame from the vertical. Normally, the tilt should not be >7°, from the vertical. But it has been observed that ill-fitting frames tilt to a larger extent, causing prismatic effect.

d. *Centering:* One of the most important issues in spectacle fitting process is the 'centration' of the lens in the frame. Ideally, the optical axis of the lens should coincide with the visual axis. In large lenses or in high number lenses, the fitting has to be modified and the lenses cut in such a manner that both the centres coincide. This principle applies most in high cylindrical fittings. If the optical centre of lens is too low or too high than the visual axis, prismatic effect causes 'jumping' of images when the eyes are moved in different directions.

e. *Vertex distance:* The vertex distance is the distance of the spectacle lens from the front of cornea. The 'effective power' of the lens changes according to the distance from the cornea.

This applies to all type of lenses, but more so in cylindrical lenses as the prismatic effect also varies with the distance.

Contact Lenses

a. *Rigid contact lenses (RGP):* Because almost all astigmatisms result from the front surface of the cornea, rigid gas-permeable lenses are an ideal solution. Since they are rigid, the lens can mould the tear film on the front surface of cornea into a spherical shape.

   RGP contact lenses can correct astigmatism without a toric design. This is possible because these lenses are 'rigid' and retain their spherical shape on the eye, instead of conforming to the toric surface of the cornea. The uniformly spherical front surface of the lens replaces the misshapen cornea as the primary refracting surface. The best use of RGP lenses is in 'irregular astigmatism', where even the toric RGP lens also does not hold good.

   There are RGP lenses with toric design, but are needed for high amounts of astigmatism. Most children appreciate crisp vision with an RGP lens, but owing to their rigid nature, adaptation takes longer and may be uncomfortable in long hours of use.

b. *Toric contact lenses:* The name stems from their unique design and are specifically used to correct astigmatism. Rigid as well as soft lenses are available in toric design. The toric lens has different curvature meridian moulded on the front surface and is placed in a particular position to correct that meridian. However, if the lens rotates, then the purpose is defeated and the vision becomes blurred. This drawback has also been overcome by installing a 'ballast' at one end of the lens, so that the lens remains stable and does not rotate.

   The soft lenses are either made of conventional hydrogel material or highly 'breathable' silicone hydrogel material. Since different companies make specific type, having different axes; one has to choose the brand that provides the best fit, comfort, and vision.

c. *Hybrid contact lenses:* These lenses have a central zone made of rigid gas-permeable material surrounded by a fitting zone of soft material. When properly fitted, hybrid contact lenses provide the best of both types of lenses, viz. a sharp, crisp vision of RGP and wearing comfort of the soft lens.

Hybrid lenses are of the same sizes as the soft lenses and have thinner edges than an RGP lens. There is less risk of these lenses getting dislodged during sports or other physical activities.

Fitting of a hybrid lens is similar to an RGP lens and takes more time and expertise than fitting a soft lens.

d. *Special contact lenses:* There was a time when choice of contact lens was very limited. Today, there are many brands and styles of contact lenses, specially toric lenses. In soft toric lenses, designs and materials are available for monthly use and throwaway—disposable lenses. Also coloured toric lenses are available which serve the cosmetic purpose also. To add to the basket, 'toric bifocal lenses' are available which correct presbyopia also. Toric silicone hydrogel lenses, which are designed for 'extended wear use', can be worn for up to 30 days overnight.

'Proclear multifocal toric lens' is a good example of a bifocal toric lens. There are some more companies making lenses with their own trade name, as the book will not venture into the commercial aspect, it cannot be further described.

Corneal Collagen Crosslinking

The mechanism of action of this special type of treatment is by strengthening and increasing the collagen crosslinks of cornea which are the 'natural anchors' of the cornea. These anchors keep the cornea in its proper shape and prevent it from bulging or changing its shape.

The procedure consists of saturating the cornea with custom-made riboflavin drops, which is then activated by ultraviolet light. This further strengthens the crosslinking of the corneal collagen.

Laser treatment of cornea: This is similar to treatment of myopia, and has been already described.

Points to note

As we know, astigmatism, like any other refractive error, is either hereditary or acquired. The first cause cannot be prevented; while the second cause can be controlled to some extent. There are certain points given below which presumably have a bearing on the progression of certain types of refractive error, especially astigmatism.

1. Certain diseases of the eyes, particularly allergic disorders of eyes, lid abnormalities, skin diseases, have been associated with astigmatism. Long-standing tumors of the lids, inflammatory or otherwise, have been known to propagate astigmatism.

2. Continuous rigorous rubbing of eyes, as in cases of vernal kerato-conjunctivitis, has been associated with progression of astigmatism and keratoconus.

3. Deficiency, particularly of vitamin A and vitamin D, has been anecdotally blamed for astigmatism, probably owing to its effect on cornea.

Amblyopia

HISTORY

The history of amblyopia is a fascinating one that vividly demonstrates how its concepts influenced the handling of the disease. Le Cat in 1713 provided the first accurate clinical description of human amblyopia. He described dull vision in an eye which apparently looked normal.

However, the credit of first describing treatment of amblyopia goes to a French naturalist and botanist Comte De Buffon (1707–1788). Buffon was first to realize the two most important elements of amblyopia therapy, viz. occlusion and optical correction. Though the principles of occlusion were not described, what was clearly observed was the improvement in vision with spectacles.

However, occlusion of one eye is supposed to be described much earlier by Thabiti-bin-Qurrah, whose date of birth is not known but died in AD 900. This scientist and philosopher from Mesopotamia wrote that "squinting should be treated by patching of the good eye". Once this is done, the visual power of the good eye will go in entirety to the deviated eye and vision will be restored in that eye. He continues to write that "such patients should also be purged; should bathe every second day, and should be made to sneeze by putting olive oil in the nose". His second writing seems to be difficult to digest but so also is doubtful whether the concept of patching existed at that time.

Nevertheless, from wherever this idea originated at that time, this principle of amblyopia therapy has remained virtually unchanged for more than a millennium!

Despite these early recommendations, amblyopia was not treated for a long time. Indeed, treatment was rejected as amblyopia was thought to be a congenital, hereditary anomaly for which no treatment existed. This view continued until 1935, when S. Gifford reported from Chicago that he reinvented patching but the results were not consistent. Chavasse in 1939 tried to describe the dull vision due to certain factors in early childhood. He observed a large number of children who had difficulty in seeing, also had refractive errors and deviation of eyes. Prescribing spectacles improved vision in many children but not all. He concluded that those who had refractive errors from very early childhood responded less to optical correction than who developed visual defect later. He thus conceived the theory of 'amblyopia of arrest' versus 'amblyopia of extinction'. Banking on this concept, Debson and Teller in 1978, hypothesized that 'amblyopia of arrest' can only exist when the abnormal visual experience develops before 6 months of age. The majority of amblyopia is of 'extinction' type and is reversible.

With the birth of the concept that amblyopia is a sensory defect of strabismus and not a congenital one, patching was resumed and has since remained the mainstay of treatment.

Attempts were made to supplement the passive patching treatment with active stimulation of the poor eye. Electrical, chemical, photogenic therapies were tried without success.

Certain visual exercises to train the amblyopic eye were also suggested. All these did not yield the desirable satisfactory results. Alfred Bangerter in 1960s introduced active stimulation of the fovea by a method called 'Pleoptics'. Notwithstanding the test of time, these measures faded into oblivion.

For the last 50 years, vast number of eminent clinicians and researchers have tried to explain the etiopathogenesis or pathophysiology of amblyopia. Tilldate, we are still unaware of the exact site or location of the pathology, how to reverse it or prevent it! The management itself, unfortunately, has not progressed beyond what was available decades ago. Even the definition of amblyopia is not clear!

As amblyopia is the most common cause of unilateral visual disability, it needs more attention. We shall see into the following pages that more we dig deeper into the mystery of amblyopia, the more we get intrigued!

Definitions

Amblyopia in Greek means 'dull vision'. The following definitions are used commonly and are interchangeable. All convey the same meaning, but differently:

a. "Amblyopia can be defined as a reduction in visual acuity with no demonstrable abnormality in the eye" (Christine Powell and Sarah Hatt, 2008).

b. "Best corrected visual acuity in one or both eyes not improving than 6/9; or a difference of more than 2 Snellen chart line in eyes with the best optical correction with no pathology detected in the eyes".

c. Others defined amblyopia as "Reduced visual acuity in the eye or eyes without any ophthalmoscopically detectable anomaly in the eye".

Traditionally, amblyopia has been defined as "Decrease in best corrected vision for which no cause can be detected by physical examination of the eyes, and caused by vision deprivation or abnormal binocular interaction" (Von Noorden, 1996).

Amblyopia does not only affect the visual acuity (recognition acuity), but also vernier acuity, contrast sensitivity, stereoacuity, and dark adaptations. All the above visual functions are concurrently decreased depending on the degree of amblyopia. Stereoacuity, in particular, goes hand-in-hand with the visual acuity.

Two very pertinent questions arise with all the traditional definitions: First, visual acuity is not the only visual function affected in amblyopia, as all definitions consider the visual acuity as the parameter of definition; and second, the words—"no pathology or abnormality seen in eyes" is misleading, as in 'deprivation amblyopia', there is always a pathology in the eye in the visual axis, which hampers the formation of clear, distinct image on the fovea. Congenital cataracts, corneal opacities, vitreous opacities, etc. are all known causes of deprivation amblyopia, and these are all pathologies in the eye.

Therefore, the definition of amblyopia needs to be redefined and reconstructed. "Amblyopia, in strict sense, is a combination of many decreased visual functions, caused by a myriad of abnormalities in the eye, which affect the normal development of visual pathways and the visual cortex".

Any disorder of the eye which interferes with the normal 'neurovisual' development should be a part of the definition of amblyopia. In fact, amblyopia is a syndrome of abnormal or 'arrested neurovisual development' caused by any disorder in the eye which interferes with formation of a clear, sharp image on the fovea. Majority of definitions stress on the visual acuity only, but in studying amblyopia, other visual functions should be taken into account.

EPIDEMIOLOGY

According to general consensus, the prevalence of amblyopia is between 3 and 5% in the general population. The distribution of mild to moderate amblyopia as per the etiology in children is anisometropic 38%, strabismic 37%, and mixed 24%. That means, the incidence is almost equally distributed in all three groups of etiology.

In severe amblyopias, the incidence of 'mixed' cause rises to 38%. In older children, the prevalence in strabismic and mixed amblyopia drops down; while the incidence of anisometropic amblyopia rises.

The reason is simple as anisometropia goes undetected for a long time; whereas strabismic patients tend to report much earlier.

A recent data regarding prevalence of amblyopia at age 7–8 years is provided by AVON Longitudinal Studies of parents and children in a UK based cohort study. Of the 6000 children assessed, 16.7% had undergone preschool vision screening and all children were offered vision screening at school entry (age

5 years). The prevalence of amblyopia was twice in children who underwent vision screening late than who underwent at the 'preschool age'. These data were confirmed by a similar study in Israel, which found 1.0% amblyopia in older children previously screened as 'preschool testing' and taken amblyopia treatment as compared to 3.0% amblyopia who had not received any treatment. These findings confirm a very important aspect of amblyopia that early detection at preschool level or at school entry level by visual screening has a huge potential in detecting the risk factors of amblyopia and their subsequent early treatment.

PATHOPHYSIOLOGY OF AMBLYOPIA

Amblyopia is a developmental disorder of the neurovisual system. It is caused by abnormal visual experience during early childhood, and results in persistent deficits in cortical processing, even when normal visual inputs to the visual cortex are restored.

In all types of amblyopia, the 'fundus' has been found to be absolutely normal. Apparently no abnormality has been found at the retina or nerve–head level. Thus it has long been conceived that the problem lies far ahead in the visual pathways and beyond. Electrophysiological, radioisotope, and autopsy studies of amblyopic patients have convincingly proved that the defects lie in the lateral geniculate body, the primary visual cortex and areas extending beyond the primary visual cortex!

From a neurologic scientific perspective, experimentally induced amblyopia is one of the most widely used animal models for investigating the mechanisms underlying visual cortex development and plasticity.

David Hubel and Toresten Weisel won the Nobel Prize in physiology in 1981 for their work in showing the extent of damage to 'ocular dominant columns' in kittens by sufficient visual deprivation during the so-called 'critical period' of visual development. The part of brain receiving images from the affected eye is not stimulated properly and does not develop to its full functional potential. This revelation opened the mystery of complex processes in the brain regarding vision development during early years and may be even later! (*see* Chapter 2 on Neural Maturation). Animal models of amblyopia allow for the role of sensory experience in cortical development to be explored, and enable investigations into the ability of environmental and pharmacological manipulations to induce neuroplasticity in the brain.

Amblyopia is also relevant to cognitive neuroscience as human amblyopia provides important insights into the role of co-ordinated, binocular experience in the vision development. Indeed psychophysical studies of amblyopia have revealed a broad range of visual deficits associated with amblyopia which are not limited to visual acuity and binocular function only. These can be loosely grouped into 'impaired perception' within the visual scene (local processing), and deficits affecting the integration of multiple elements across space and time and can be called 'global processing'. Impaired local processing is often linked to abnormalities within the primary visual cortex (V1), containing cells which tend to have relatively small receptive fields. Global processing impairments, on the other hand, are thought to involve extra-striate areas (cortical areas V5–V6). These areas tend to have larger receptive fields and integrate signals emanating from other areas of visual pathways.

A hypothesis proposed by Van Essen and Gallan in 1994, says that extra-striate visual areas are specialized in representing the location and movements of objects across space and, therefore, provide a foundation of visuo-motor co-ordination. This processing pathway is also referred to as 'dorsal' or 'vision for action' and extends from occipital to parietal lobe.

The second pathway, known as the 'ventral' or 'vision for recognition', includes ventral regions of the occipital and temporal lobes and is thought to be specialized for processing of 'form' which includes object recognition. This processing hypothesis has provided a useful framework for the investigation of global processing in visual development and amblyopia (Simmers, et al. 2006).

While it is now well accepted that amblyopia results in deficits far beyond the central vision, a key question still remains: Are the deficits in extra-striate areas pertaining to motion of objects, their relative motions, hand–eye co-ordinations, the ability to recall, etc. simply an extention of local processing defects (defects in the primary visual cortex, area V1) or far fetched deficits impaired independently by faulty visual inputs? Answering this question will provide important insights into the role of sensory experience in the cortical development, plasticity and the visual impairment experienced by patients with amblyopia.

Amblyopia is primarily thought of as a disorder of spatial vision, as reflected by the clinical emphasis on reduced visual acuity. Clinical research and studies on patients have shown that amblyopia affects multiple aspects of vision including contrast sensitivity, hyperacuity (vernier acuity), crowding, colour vision, stereoacuity, and spatial processing—which broadly means recognition of position in space, motion, hand-eye coordination, visual memory and recall.

The most significant affect of amblyopia other than visual acuity is on contrast sensitivity, stereoacuity, hyperacuity and crowding—which are addressed by the primary visual cortex. Hyperacuity refers to the ability to detect spatial details that are beyond the resolution of the cone photoreceptors. An example is the vernier acuity, whereby persons are able to identify offsets in alignments that are smaller in visual angle than the resolution limit of retina. Crowding refers to impaired recognition or detection of a target object when it is flanked by distractions. For example, a letter presented in isolation in the visual field is better recognized than a letter 'crowded' or 'surrounded' by adjacent letters or bars. Patients with strabismic amblyopia have been found to exhibit impaired vernier acuity and crowding in central vision. Similar deficits have been reported in anisometropic amblyopia, but the defects are less pronounced.

Contrast sensitivity is reduced in all forms of amblyopia. In deprivation amblyopia, the impairment is much severe, more pronounced in unilateral than bilateral cases. However, the extent of impairment is strongly tied to the duration of deprivation and age of onset.

The current literature suggests that a difference of blur between the eyes (anisometropia) during the development period creates less impairment in functions related to extra-striate areas than strabismic amblyopia. This proves the importance of binocularity in such type of amblyopia (McKee, et al. 2003). In a large study which included patients of all three categories of amblyopia, it was found that persons with strabismic amblyopia (deprived of binocular function) exhibited greater losses in optotype and vernier acuity, while crowding problem and stereoacuity is affected in aniso-metropic, strabismic and mixed types of amblyopia.

Together, these studies suggest that binocular inputs strongly support the development of area V1 of the visual cortex. The effects of deprivation amblyopia on the above visual functions have not been precisely investigated. However, measurable binocular function is rare in both unilateral and bilateral deprivation amblyopias, particularly when it is congenital and addressed late. This confirms that simultaneously optotype acuity and crowding phenomena are also equally affected.

Contrast sensitivity is affected more in strabismic amblyopia than anisometropic amblyopia. Understanding of deprivation amblyopia is limited as it is related to number of factors stated above.

Broadly speaking, contrast sensitivity is affected in all forms of amblyopia, with severity in accordance to the optotype visual acuity status.

The other areas which are affected by amblyopia are the understanding of motion and relative motion. Sensitivity to motion is present throughout the visual pathways; however, the accurate representation of complex moving objects often requires integration across extended regions of visual field. Primary visual cortex (area V1) signals incoherent motion and it has been proposed that cells within the dorsal extrastriate regions of visual cortex such as area V5 in humans, integrate these signals to reconstruct the pattern of motion of these moving objects. Amblyopia thus affects the understanding to perceive the movements of objects across the visual field by its direct effect on the primary visual cortex. To perceive the movement of single object or relative movements of multiple objects across the space has important bearing in daily life as we move about and ironically this deficiency can jeopardize our movements!

Similar to motion, 'form perception' is also an integrated work of several visual areas. Evidence from animal electro-physiology (Connor, 2001 and Nandy, et al. 2013) and human MRI studies (Connor, 2007) suggest that integration of recognizing 'form' involves the areas V2 and V4, the neurons of which deal with complex form information of sizes and shapes of objects. Somehow, these functions get affected in cases of deep amblyopias, probably because of integration of these areas with the primary visual cortex.

The practical implication of 'vision of motion' is of immense importance in our daily life. When an object approaches towards us or when we cross a railway track, the relative motion of us and the coming train must be accurately gauged; similarly while crossing a busy road, the speeds of oncoming cars must be gauged; failing which we are prone to accidents. Similar examples apply to playing games, where motion in real time is affected because of amblyopia. Let's see an astonishing revelation in amblyopia. A number of studies have reported widespread processing deficits for 'both eyes' of patients with unilateral amblyopia, strongly implicating abnormalities affecting 'binocular' regions of striate and extrastriate visual cortices. This effect is reported more for 'motion' than 'form' recognizing tasks. Although less widely studied, patients with bilateral deprivation amblyopia understandably, appear to perform more poorly than unilateral deprivation amblyopia. Studies of experimental modules like monkeys, which are closest to humans, have revealed non-functional areas in the visual cortex. Demmer et al demonstrated significant reduced blood flow and oxygen uptake during visual stimulation of the amblyopic eye during 'positron emission tomography scan'. Also, the ocular dominance columns in the striate visual cortex (area V1) associated with the amblyopic eye were shown to be markedly 'attenuated' in monkeys. One important point to be understood is the difference between 'diplopia' and 'confusion'.

Diplopia results when two 'different' parts of retina visualize the 'same' object, but their visual axes are directed in different directions in space (image falling on two disparate points in retina); 'confusion' results when the two 'fovea' visualize two different objects in space. In anisometropic and deprivation amblyopias, the defocused or blurred image in one eye is not accepted in the visual cortex as it does not match with the clear, well-focused image of the other eye and is, therefore, 'suppressed'. It is here that 'inhibitory' impulses from the good eye monocular cells in the visual cortex play a role in creating amblyopia in the affected eye. In strabismic amblyopia, the image is formed at totally disparate or different parts of retina. The retinal image on the deviated eye, by virtue of not falling on the fovea, is so indistinct that it is neglected. At the same time, a state of 'confusion' also ensues, as the fovea of the deviated eye is pointing at a dissimilar object in space and this image is immediately suppressed. 'Suppression' of the foveal image of the deviated eye and 'indistinct' image from the extra-foveal part, both contribute to causation of amblyopia. In certain extraordinary situations, the sensory adaptation in some children may be so strong that the extra-foveal part of retina of the deviated eye assumes the function of fovea, 'eccentric fixation' results in monocular viewing and 'anomalous retinal correspondence' in binocular viewing.

Summary

The inference from all the studies and research derived is that abnormal visual inputs is the root cause of disturbance in the normal development of the visual pathways and the visual cortex. Therefore, a clear, crisp, distinct retinal image of the object is a prerequisite to normal development of the visual cortex and related areas. A blurred, distorted image may emerge from any of the reasons stated. Furthermore, in cases of uniocular causes, the impairment is more severe, probably because the brain relies heavily on the visual input from the good eye; in addition, to avoid confusion, the image is further suppressed by 'inhibitory' impulses dispatched to the area reserved for monocular vision in the visual cortex of the affected eye.

RISK FACTORS IN AMBLYOPIA

On an average, 40–60% of children with anisometropia and/ or strabismus in childhood will develop amblyopia. Incidence is 2–4% in the general population. Amblyopia is essentially a developmental disorder, as the same conditions responsible for amblyopia in childhood, has no lasting effect on vision when it occurs in adulthood. Therefore, there lies a 'critical period' for the development of amblyopia. Experience suggests that 'amblyogenic age' does not extend beyond 7 years of age! But the severity of disorder is linked to the age of onset. Research has shown that a 'critical period' to cause irreversible damage is 0–6 months of age. It is also known that surprisingly, there are different critical periods to affect different visual functions.

The other important risk factors which play a role in the pathogenesis of amblyopia are family history, uncorrected refractive errors, poorly corrected refractive errors, strabismus, media opacities. Any condition in early childhood like Down's syndrome, Duane's syndrome, orbital maldevelopmental disorders, craniofacial dysostosis and similar conditions which hamper the proper alignment of eyes, are all risk factors for amblyopia.

TYPES OF AMBLYOPIA

1. *Anisometropic amblyopia:* This type of amblyopia is probably the most common type or is encountered most frequently owing to a simple reason that most of times, it is detected far too late in life. Anisometropia of any kind is liable to produce amblyopia. Hyperopic anisometropia has more potential to produce the disorder than myopic anisometropia.

   Any spherical discrepancy of more than 1 dioptre between the two eyes (specially hyperopic) can potentially create amblyopia; and any discrepancy of even 0.75 D cylindrical difference between the two eyes, can produce amblyopia.

Points to note _____ •••■■

A very important pearl to be kept in mind is that when a person comes with diminution of vision in one eye, and does not yield fruitful result with best of spectacle correction, even with a seemingly small unilateral refractive error, amblyopia must be kept in mind. *The reason is simple:* This patient with a small 0.5 or 0.75 cylinder or plus 1 hyperopia, which seems innocuous today, but had a refractive error of more than 'plus' 2 or more unilaterally, which has decreased with time, but has left with a permanent amblyopic deficiency of vision!

2. *Strabismic:* Misalignment of eyes or strabismus is the next most common type of amblyogenic factor for amblyopia. Esotropia, which occurs very early in life, has more potency to cause severe amblyopia. Exotropias usually appear late in childhood, and cause less severe type of amblyopia.

3. *Mixed type:* This type comprises of strabismic and aniso-metropic cause of amblyopia; and is the third common type.

4. *Deprivation amblyopia:* This type of amblyopia is less common and occurs when the visual axis of the eye is obstructed by some pathology like cataract, corneal opacity, vitreous opacities, PHPV, etc.

   Deprivation results in more severe amblyopia because most of times they are congenital; and obscure the visual axis during the most crucial time of visual development.

   Apart from these common types of amblyopia, there are some other less common types of amblyopia but must be known and understood.

5. *Ametropic amblyopia:* It is a type of bilateral amblyopia where both eyes have same or equal refractive error, but the amount of refractive error is so high, that the visual system of eyes has difficulty in creating a clear, distinct image on the retina.

6. *Reverse or occlusion amblyopia:* It is basically an iatrogenic amblyopia, where uncontrolled, prolonged, patching of the good eye has been done, resulting in amblyopia in the previously better eye.

7. *Pathological amblyopia:* Pathological amblyopia generally does not fit into the domain of true amblyopia, as the defect or pathology is in the retina itself. Any pathology in early childhood in the retina/macular area where image has not

formed or has not given any normal visual input to the visual cortex, and thus has virtually created a deprivation type of condition and deep amblyopia in addition to the original deficit.

CLINICAL FEATURES

Anisometropic amblyopia, unfortunately, goes unnoticed for a long time. Either it is discovered accidentally, or discovered during eye checkup at school or at a clinic. In contrast, strabismic or mixed amblyopia is detected quite early owing to its obvious disposition. Deprivation amblyopia stands somewhere in between. Secondary deviations and a white reflex in the pupil are the hallmarks for detection of amblyopia in these cases. In context of management, amblyopia is divided into mild, moderate and severe. The subjective symptoms in anisometropic amblyopia, are minimal. The patient may complain of 'asthenopia'. These also occur only if the good eye has some refractive error. By and large, diminished vision, detected suddenly by the patient is a classical symptom.

Apart from visual acuity, the following other visual functions are affected:

1. *Grating acuity:* Grating acuity is the most basic visual function. As already described in the Chapter on Visual Evaluation, it is well developed from infancy itself. Any impediment to the normal development of vision in early infancy will affect the grating acuity. Timely intervention will revive this function to its full potential.

2. *Vernier acuity:* This is a high level of acuity of vision, also sometimes referred to as 'hyperacuity'. This is a function of the visual cortex, far beyond the scope of retinal fovea. With the brunt of the injury falling on visual cortex, this function is affected.

3. *Contrast sensitivity:* Contrast sensitivity, as mentioned already, is the function of the visual system to identify an object from its surroundings or background. Contrast sensitivity will be affected in all types of amblyopia and is a strong measure of the depth of amblyopia.

4. *Accommodation:* Accommodative amplitude is conspicuously affected, and is directly proportional to the severity of amblyopia. Severely amblyopic eyes do not accommodate; and this point must be kept in mind when prescribing glasses for treatment of amblyopia. Initially full correction has to be given; as the amblyopic eye improves and accommodation is restored, then the full correction can be weaned. But care should be taken in cases of high levels of anisometropia, because after the completion of ambyopia therapy, these eyes are prone to slip back into amblyopia and a controlled correction is warranted. This will be dealt in more detail in treatment part of this chapter.

5. *Afferent pupillary defect:* Afferent pupillary defect (APD), as is commonly known, is one of important features in the clinical examination. The exact nature of this defect is not clearly known but is thought to be due to poor afferent impulses reaching the midbrain area. Except in very severe amblyopias, it is difficult to establish the APD. A point to be noted here is that since there is suppression scotoma at the fovea, any light falling around it will exhibit a good pupillary reaction. For elicitation of a poor or normal pupillary response, a pencil beam of light should fall straight on the fovea. This is Stilles-Crawford effect, but is difficult to execute. Nevertheless, severe amblyopias do elicit an APD, and is a good indicator of the severity of the disease.

6. *Unsteady fixation:* Steady fixation to any object is a hallmark of good visual acuity. Poor or unsteady fixation, along with poor maintenance of fixation towards object during slow pursuit movement, is another important sign of amblyopia. At the same time, objects may be lost out of sight in space while tracking them or their tracking may be inaccurate.

7. *Stereopsis:* One of the most significant clinical signs of amblyopia is the loss of stereopsis. The gravity of loss depends upon the severity of the disorder. In severe cases, the stereopsis may drop down to 800 to 1000 seconds of arc. Stereoacuity in a normal person averages around 40 seconds of arc. As the visual acuity improves, there is a concomitant improvement in the stereoacuity also. Delay in treatment of

amblyopia, or even after successful improvement in visual acuity, some persons lack any measurable stereopsis.

8. *Adaptations:* Binocular adaptations like deep suppression, eccentric fixation, and abnormal retinal correspondence, develop in many cases of long-standing amblyopias.

EVALUATION OF AMBLYOPIA

1. *Visual acuity:* Conventionally, there should be at least 2-line difference (Snellen optotype or ETDRS chart) between the two eyes with the best optical correction. If refractive error is doubted, then age appropriate cycloplegic drug should be used and post-cycloplegic (**not post-mydriatic**) test should be performed to establish the best corrected vision. It is to be noted that mydriasis comes first and wanes off also earlier than cycloplegia. If unhurried post-cycloplegic correction yields a 2-line difference between the two eyes, then amblyopia should be suspected.

2. *Afferent pupillary defect:* APD, as already discussed above, an amblyopic eye may show subtle difference in the direct pupillary reaction of the two eyes.

3. *Crowding phenomenon:* An amblyopic eye faces difficulty in reading optotypes in a linear fashion (continues words in a line) or if the letters are 'flanked' from sides. Thus single letters are more easily read and spelled than letters surrounded by other letters. This 'crowding phenomenon' is a unique clinical feature in amblyopia, and should be always kept in mind while evaluating.

4. *Neutral density filter:* Neutral density (ND) filters are made of glass, which reduce or modify all wavelengths of light (colours) equally. They are extensively used in photography. In ophthalmology, they are used to identify amblyopia and distinguish between functional and organic amblyopia. They come as colourless and in shades of grey. It has been found that using an ND filter in front of amblyopic eye, further reduces the visual acuity by approximately 2 lines; while in non-amblyopic eyes, the reduction may be negligible (Fig. 7.1).

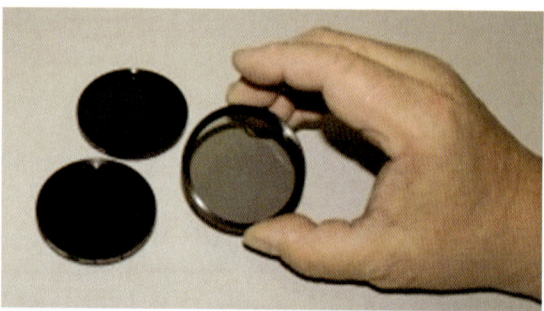

Fig. 7.1: Neutral density filters of various shades

5. *Worth's four-dot test:* This is an excellent method of defining amblyopia severity. An area of central suppression will be found with the Worth test. Comparison between distance and near Worth four-dot test will also show the extent of area of central suppression.

6. *Prism test:* A prism of 4 to 6 PD, base down, if placed in front of non-amblyopic eye, will promote an upward shift of both eyes. But such a prism placed in front of amblyopic eye will not usher any drift in either eye.

7. *Vanishing vision:* Typically, when testing visual acuity by Snellen chart, the patient experiences that some part of letter becomes visible then disappears, then some other part of letter becomes visible. This creates confusion in distinguishing that particular letter (Fig. 7.2).

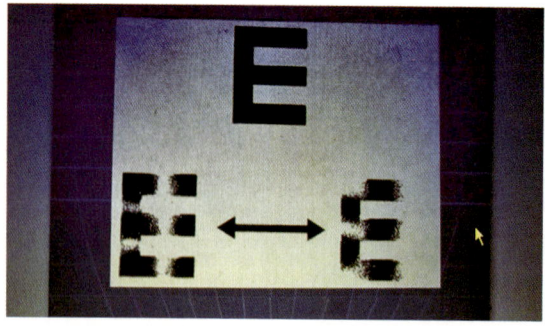

Fig. 7.2: Letter distortions in an amblyope

8. *Fundus examination:* This is the ultimate test to verify amblyopia. As per the traditional definitions, the fundus of the amblyopic eye will show no pathology.

9. *Cycloplegic refraction:* Cycloplegic refraction, with age matched cycloplegic drug, is the front runner in diagnosing refractive error as a cause of certain types of refractive error-induced amblyopias. It is to be noted that a spherical anisometropia of even 1.25 D and astigmatic difference of 0.75 D, between the two eyes, is enough to produce amblyopia.

MANAGEMENT OF AMBLYOPIA

As already explained in previous pages, amblyopia encompasses multiple visual defects, all triggered by abnormal or improper visual input to the visual cortex. These defects are not only limited to the primary visual cortex, (area V1), but affect other cortical areas also (area V2, V4, V5, V6), which deal with integration and execution of other visual functions.

Unfortunately, all these defects occur in the early ages of development, when detection is difficult and is usually missed, though a subset of amblyopia patients have shown improvement in adult age also. Most of these defects can be corrected successfully by timely detection and treatment but treatment delay leaves a permanent mark.

Critical Period

There has been a lot of speculation about the 'critical period' of visual development. There are known different critical periods for different deficits but all researchers agree that age 0–6 months is the most crucial for rapid neurovisual development. Any type of image disturbance or disruption during this period leaves a lasting impact, even after the normal input is restored. Binocularity develops between 4 and 6 months of age; vernier acuity, hand–eye coordination, vision for motion, which require binocular vision as a prerequisite, are affected, if the binocular vision is not restored by this period. Visual acuity or grating acuity establishes itself quite early in life, by 3 months.

Recognition acuity (optotype vision) continues to mature up to 5 years of age. A great deal depends upon the 'plasticity ' or the 'recovery power' of the brain. Enormous research is now ongoing to understand the plasticity of various regions of the brain, and the neurotransmitters which govern them. We shall review them in detail in later pages of this chapter.

Most studies and clinicians believe that the visual cortex has matured sufficiently by the age 7–8 years, and any obstacle to vision after this period, does not produce amblyopia. Thus 0–8 years is termed as the 'amblyogenic age'. But it must be borne in mind that amblyopia 'reverts' back in many cases, even after a successful treatment. Therefore, the patient has to be kept under surveillance at least up to 12 years of age, and I personally keep the patient under surveillance for up to 14 years of age. This points towards a fact that though severity may be less, but amblyogenic age may prolong up to 12 years also.

Prognosis of Treatment

The prognosis of treatment of any type of amblyopia rests on many factors, which are narrated as follows:

1. *Age of onset:* Perhaps this is the most crucial factor. Congenital or infantile tropia or any impediment in the visual axis at this age bears the worst prognosis, if not treated in time. Critical period of visual development is most relevant here.

2. *Type of amblyopia:* Anisometropia, strabismus and deprivation, all have the propensity to cause amblyopia of any severity. Unfortunately, unilateral refractive error is not detected early and becomes refractory to treatment in later ages.

   Manifest strabismus and deprivation due to congenital cataract present early, and have better prognosis, if managed properly.

3. *Severity of amblyopia:* Another significant factor in gauging prognosis is the severity or depth of amblyopia. Severity is inversely proportional to the outcome of treatment.

4. *Duration of amblyopia:* Lesser the duration of amblyopia, the better prognosis it carries. Long-standing amblyopias, and amblyopia detected late in life are more refractory to treatment and thus carry poor prognosis.

5. *Time of intervention:* It goes without saying that early the diagnosis and initiation of treatment, better the outcome. Manifest congenital tropia, or tropia secondary to congenital cataract and a congenital corneal opacity are no doubt detected quite early, but their expert management is lacking in most centres, and therefore, bear a bad prognosis because of untimely or improper management.

6. *Compliance to treatment:* One of the major issues to the success of treatment is poor compliance. Patching, which is the mainstay of treatment, is usually not followed in letter and spirit. Clinical experience has shown that patching is done less than the hours prescribed.

   Schoolgoing children object to patching during school hours or remove the patch while in school. Parents too succumb to the wishes of their wards, and do not adhere to the schedule.

   Moreover, the follow-up schedule is not religiously maintained. Spectacles are improperly worn with slipping on nose or tilting, a common problem; lenses are untidy or full of scratches. All these are hindrances to the success of treatment.

7. *Associated anomalies:* Besides the ocular problem, there are other neuropsychological disorders which also contribute to the poor compliance to treatment. Children with mental defects or retardation, delayed milestones, premature births, etc. are a large group where the success of treatment is guarded.

Aim of Amblyopia Therapy

The basic strategy of treatment is to create a clear, sharp image on the retinal fovea and promote the use of the amblyopic eye.

Clarity of image is achieved by eliminating the causative factor of blurred image. And then the amblyopic eye is forced to work by blocking the vision in the good eye. Blocking the normal eye and the formation of clear, distinct image on the retina, sends positive impulses to the monocular cells in the brain—which so far have been dormant; and also stops the inhibitory impulses to the visual cortex representing the amblyopic eye from the normal eye, and reverses the pathology in the lateral geniculate body and the visual cortex.

Treatment Options

The following modes of treatment are available for the management of amblyopia:

1. Occlusion of the good eye.
2. Medical penalization of the good eye.
3. Optical penalization of the good eye.
4. Active stimulation of the amblyopic eye.

Let us discuss each one of them. It is to be remembered that the visual axis has to be cleared and a sharp, focused image formed on the retina before any mode of therapy is instituted.

Occlusion Therapy

Occlusion or totally blocking vision of the sound eye by suitable material has been the mainstay of treatment for amblyopia for decades. This has stood the test of time and very little has changed in this mode over the time.

The standard, conventional way is to 'occlude' the sound eye totally with a 'patch'. The patch is like a sticker, adhering to the skin on the closed eyelids, thus fully and completely blocking any visual stimuli reaching the retina. The amblyopic eye is now forced to work. It is of paramount importance that a clear, well-defined image should be presented to the fovea. This, over time, stimulates the process of normalization of the visual pathways and the primary visual cortex and consequently the improvement in vision.

A number of studies have deduced a formula to determine the 'regime of patching' as follows:

a. From birth to one year of age—one hour of patching per month of age, but not more than six hours of constant patch.
b. From one year to twelve years—one week per year of age.

This states that for an infant of 2 months, daily patching of 2 hours is optimum; and for an infant of 8 months, maximum of 6 hours of patch is sufficient. This should be strictly followed to avoid the risk of 'reverse' amblyopia. Reverse amblyopia is an iatrogenic entity, caused by excessive patching of the sound eye.

Following the above regime, for a child of 6 years, continuous patching is advised for 6 weeks; for 8 years age, up to 8 weeks and so on. This standard regime does not always work, as there are other factors influencing amblyopia. Therefore, patching has to be titrated, i.e. the number of hours and number of weeks have to be adjusted taking into account the severity and other factors affecting amblyopia. Rule of thumb does not always apply and by large, all the factors including the compliance to treatment have to be carefully studied. Cinical experience of the author showed that with severe amblyopia, vision 6/36 and lower, patching has to be continued for a longer time, than the stipulated regime, but not longer than 6 months. The maximum response achieved is by 6 months of patching. Continuing beyond this period does not yield any extra benefit. Another aspect is the 'number of hours' of patching. Standard treatment recommends 'full waking hours' that is, 12 hours/day patching in severe cases. If the child sleeps for 2 hours during the day, then the patching has to be extended. Clinical experience has shown that in severe, long-standing amblyopias, 10–12 hours of daily patching gives the expected results. Another important aspect is that patching should not be done with 'broken regime'; nor patching should be alternating between the eyes; daily, all seven days patching of the good eye should be done. This should be followed as a regulation. Only the time period and the number of hours can be varied.

The following protocol is recommended.

For moderate to severe amblyopias:

a. Initial visual acuity is recorded with age appropriate targets at the beginning of treatment. Stereoacuity, where possible, should also be ideally recorded.

b. Patching (by a patch on the eye) is initiated for full waking hours, i.e. for 12 hours per day. The patch preferred in my practice is an 'Opticlude' by 3M company. Any similar patch can be used. But care should be taken that it totally obscures light from entering the eye.

c. Patient followed, preferably every 4 weeks. At each visit, visual acuity is recorded.

d. Patching is continued as per the regulation mentioned above. After 3 months of continuous patching, the strategy is re-assessed. If by 3 months, if no improvement in vision is recorded, then it is deduced that the amblyopia is 'refractory', and the treatment will not succeed. Also, if no further improvement occurs after 2 consecutive visits, then it is assumed that the optimum result has occurred, and the patching can now be weaned.

If the improvement continues, albeit slowly, the patching regime is not altered and is continued for 3 months more, when the full desired effect is achieved. In any case, the patching regime is then altered and weaned depending upon the age of the patient, severity of amblyopia, response to patching, and other conditions.

After completion of the initial treatment, stereoacuity is also recorded. Contrast sensitivity should also be assessed, where possible.

e. After maximal improvement in vision, patching is not abruptly stopped, but weaned according to a protocol. As per the authors' protocol, patching is reduced by 2 hours every 2 weeks; and follow up is done again every 4 weeks (monthly). If vision does not drop, then patching is stopped after 3 months.

f. The patient is then followed up every 3 months for a year. If vision remains constant, then the follow-up is extended to every 6 months. This regime is continued till the patient attains the age of 12 years.

During this period, if the vision drops, patching is reintroduced from the level it was discontinued. In the authors' practice, patching is resumed by 2 hours/day; and the patient is reviewed every month. The patching may be increased, if desirable results are not obtained after one month. This regime is continued for 3 months, with the idea that vision should remain stable for at least 3 months. If so, then occlusion is stopped and patient reviewed again after 1 month. If vision remains stable, the usual reviewing is resumed up to 12 years of age.

There are some important points to remember in the management of an amblyopia patient:

1. Every patient is a separate entity; and the management has to be titrated keeping in mind the various variables.

2. It is surprising that with two similar patients, the response to treatment varies.

   This will be further discussed in later pages of this chapter.

3. In milder types of amblyopia (VA 6/12 to 6/24), occlusion has been tried for fewer hours. In some cases, it has worked; while in some, the results were disappointing. A major problem with patching is that the advice of fewer hours, i.e. 2 or 4 hours, the compliance is even less than that, and as this does not offer the desirable result, it undermines the efficacy of treatment.

   Therefore, to circumvent this problem, the author begins with full time occlusion in every case, and the time schedule is from 8 AM to 8.0 PM; this ensures complete compliance and regularity in wearing the patch. Caution should be taken in advising full time (12 hours) in children below 5 years of age, because of risk of reverse amblyopia. In this group, the author reviews the patient every 2 weeks. This helps to observe the effect of patching on the vision of the amblyopic eye as well as the good eye.

There are various types of patch available in the market. The most useful is the 'skin coloured ' patch, as this is less obvious. Patches with coloured designs and objects may be attractive to the child; but at the same time are more eye-catching and obvious to the public which may be disturbing to the child and counterproductive (Fig. 7.3).

Variations in patching:

1. *Occlusion is misunderstood.* In the past and even today, the better eye is occluded by means of a spectacle with a black or dark glass. It may sound workable theoretically, but in

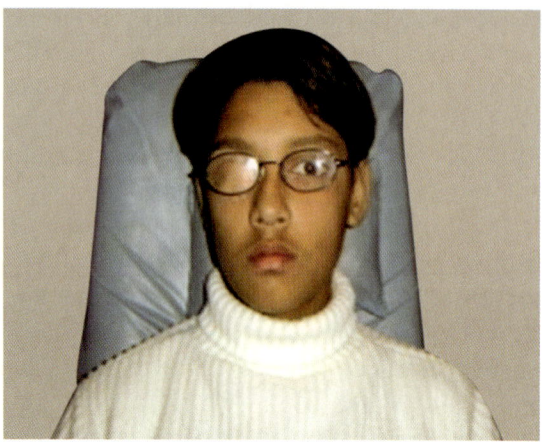

Fig. 7.3: Skin-coloured patch

fact the true principle is that the eye should be completely 'occluded' and no light should reach the retina; because even light stimulus may initiate inhibitory impulses to the visual cortical area of the amblyopic eye.

Also the probability of the child removing the specks or 'peeping' over the specks is a constant menace. As a rule, in any type of amblyopia, occlusion is the gold standard, only the time schedule may be varied.

2. *Bangerter filters:* Bangerter filters or 'foils' have been available in the market since 1960! They are translucent occluders which can be attached to the back surface of the spectacle lens and were designed as a method to modulate the degree of blurring or degrading the quality of image on the retina in the sound eye. The degree of 'degradation' of image can be predicted depending upon the type of foil used. Number 0.2 produces the least degradation. The degradation or blurring produced increases in numerical order of 0.4, 0.6, 0.8 and so on.

Bangerter foils have been mostly used as a secondary treatment or as a maintenance therapy following conventional occlusion or atropine penalization. Though they are not used now but they have *potential advantages* and thus deserve the mention:

a. The ability to modulate light by changing the density of filters is beneficial as an after-treatment for amblyopias, not as a primary treatment.

b. Better compliance and less irritating as compared to patching, as they are attached to the glass rather than the skin of the lids. This may be beneficial in recurrence of amblyopia after the conventional patching.

c. Better acceptance to the patient as they create less cosmetic blemish.

d. Less disruptive to binocular vision.

The *potential disadvantages* are:

a. As mentioned earlier, risk of patient not wearing glasses exist.

b. The child may peek around the glasses.

c. May not degrade visual acuity to the desired amount in order to stimulate the other eye.

d. May not fully comply to the specifications given by the manufacturer.

The effectiveness of the Bangerter filters as a 'primary' treatment has not been established and therefore, though available for more than half a century, have not been universally accepted.

Part time occlusion: A lot of research and speculation has been going on over the concept and efficacy of 'part-time occlusion' of the good eye. Studies in USA and elsewhere by some clinicians have shown promising results in improvement in vision of children up to 7 years of age with mild to moderate amblyopia with 2 hours of patching per day.

A PEDIG (Pediatric Eye Diseases Investigative Group, USA) study; which is a multicentric study in the United States, has shown good results in children with mild to moderate amblyopia with 4–6 hours of patching per day. (The PEDIG study has gained reputation as an authentic, broad-based study conducted by over 60 centers in the United States.)

But results in older children and severe amblyopias in younger children have not shown the desired results.

To summarize, full-time patching (10–12 hours per day) with a patch on the eye remains the gold standard for severe amblyopias, mixed amblyopias, and amblyopia in older children.

Part-time patching shows promise in younger children with mild to moderate amblyopia only. But the number of hours have to be again titrated.

In another recent PEDIG study, 2 hours patching was compared with increased number of hours patching in 170 children aged 3 to 8 years. These children underwent patching for 2 hours per day for 3 months for mild to moderate amblyopia. Improvement occurred of 3 to 4 lines on Snellen chart, but no further improvement was recorded.

These children underwent then further occlusion of 6 hours/day for further 10 weeks, when an improvement of 2 lines more was recorded.

Therefore, in author's view, part-time occlusion should be only tried in very young children as a primary therapy in mild amblyopias. If no further improvement is noticed after 3 months, then more hours of occlusion should be resorted to. Under no circumstances, treatment should be abandoned assuming that treatment is not responding.

With moderate to severe amblyopia in young children, at 6 hours/day of patching should be adopted as a primary treatment.

The duration of therapy again depends upon other factors of amblyopia prognosis.

As a rule of thumb, if vision stops improving after 2 consecutive visits of follow-up, then that is the end point of treatment; but as mentioned earlier, the therapy is weaned gradually.

In all cases, patients have to be followed initially at 6–8 weeks interval for 6 months; then at 3 months interval for 6 months; and 6 monthly up to age of 12 years. This regimen ensures a good vigilance for any relapses.

At any stage during the follow-up visits, if visual acuity drops, the patching is resumed, as discussed above.

See this example

A young girl of 11 years comes with history of diminished vision, OS, discovered accidentally.

VA-OD: 6/6; OS: 6/36.

Cyclcoplegic refraction, with cyclopentolate 1% showed:

OD: +0.5 D; OS: +2.5 CYL 90%

Obviously, the patient has severe anisometropic (meridional) amblyopia.

Treatment advised was:

1. OD patch occlusion 12 hours/day.
2. TV viewing for at least one hour.
3. Near work with fine writing/drawing to stimulate good hand–eye coordination and stereopsis.
4. Full astigmatic correction, OS.

An initial trial of spectacles, as advocated by many clinicians as a first-line management would not yield any fruitful result considering the gravity of amblyopia and age of the patient.

Points to note

Before embarking on occlusion in mild to moderate anisometropic amblyopia, it is prudent to give spectacle correction and review vision after six weeks. This six weeks of 'spectacle trial' has shown in many cases to improve vision and reduce the number of hours of occlusion.

Atropine Penalization

Atropine penalization is a method of damping the vision of the good eye, so that the amblyopic eye is forced to work. The principle is similar to occlusion albeit with advantages and some disadvantages.

Atropine is a strong parasympatholytic agent, used as drops and eye ointment to paralyze accommodation and prevent formation of well-focused image on the retina. Pupillary dilatation is an annoying concomitant effect. Severe blurring of vision is the hallmark for use of atropine over other cyclo-plegic drugs.

Atropine is used as atropine sulphate in 1% drops or ointment. The normal regime is one drop of 1% atropine sulphate daily at night, placed in the lower fornix of the good eye, with the canaliculus blocked for one minute. Atropine penalization is not used in infants and very young children owing to the fear of 'reverse amblyopia', as the good eye is 'pharmaceutically occluded' for full 24 hours, which is not desired in infants.

There is a controversy regarding the dose and schedule of atropine therapy. Some researchers advocate thrice or even twice weekly schedule, stating that this is enough to maintain total cycloplegia. Homatropine 2% can also be used, where atropine causes side effects or allergic symptoms.

Whatever drug is used for penalization, the sole purpose is to produce total cycloplegia so that the vision of the good eye remains blurred sufficiently for all distances. To meet this end, homatropine 2% or cyclopentolate 2% will have to be used more frequently. Also in young children or children with dark iris, these will not be optimally effective.

The *advantages* of atropine penalization are:
1. Causes complete cycloplegia and severe blurring of vision, and hence comparable in effectivity to patch occlusion.
2. Compliance problem is minimized.
3. Both eyes are open, so binocularity is not compromised.
4. Cosmetic blemish is not present. This adds to the compliance guarantee.
5. Good alternative to patching in mild amblyopia and during recurrences.

Disadvantages:
1. Not advisable in infants and very young children.
2. Allergic reactions are common.
3. Risk of toxic reactions in inadvertent overdosing or in idiosyncratic patients.
4. Severe photophobia.

Optical Penalization

Another way of occluding the vision is to use high power plus lens to fog the image in the good eye. This may seem very attractive option, but it has greater disadvantages. Firstly, the compliance is highly doubtful as the child can easily remove glasses at will; secondly, wearing a heavy lens on one eye is difficult and cosmetically unacceptable.

Though the problem of heavy glass lenses has to quite an extent overcome by replacing glass by plastic lens, but they cause bigger cosmetic blemish being much thicker at the edges than glass. In any case, use of a plus lens as high as + 8 to + 10.0 D in one eye makes the spectacle frame thicker and unbalanced. Most importantly, the eye is still receives full light and some degraded image, which goes against the principles of total occlusion.

Optical penalization is not used nowadays as a treatment of amblyopia.

To summarize, occlusion of the good eye by a 'patch' on the skin of the lids still remains the gold standard of modern treatment. Controversy exists regarding the number of hours of patching, but this is overcome by prudent titrating of the hours taking into account all the variable factors of amblyopia.

Bangerter foils or 'dark glasses' over the better eye, have not proved to be effective, and are not practiced as a standard protocol of amblyopia management.

Parents and patients should be counselled properly about the pros and cons of several forms of treatment available but the best suited to the type of amblyopia should be instituted. Care should be taken not to insist on patching only, allowing the option of choice of 'best tolerated' mode of therapy. Compliance is the key to success and they should be informed that the course of treatment is prolonged and follow-up is long.

Active Stimulation

Active stimulation of the retina was a modality conceived to stimulate the fovea by external means. Several authors used different techniques to stimulate the fovea by flashes of light, a practice known as *pleoptics*.

But it soon dawned that it is the 'form' of the spatial object required to stimulate the visual cortex, not light per se. Further, the retina is not the harbinger of the anomaly. Pleoptics has now been largely abandoned and newer methods of active stimulation have emerged—all aiming at stimulating the visual cortex.

Functional Impact of Amblyopia Therapy

Apart from the visual acuity, the effect of amblyopia treatment on the following visual functions also needs to be assessed.

a. *Stereoacuity:* Stereoacuity is more severely affected in strabismic amblyopia than anisometropic amblyopia. The improvement in stereoacuity, after a successful amblyopia treatment, coincides well with the improvement in visual acuity. There is evidence that some lag in the stereopsis in strabismic amblyopia remains even after complete recovery of vision. Stereoacuity in children is best tested by Frisby Davis distance and near tests. The more rapid improvement in visual acuity, the better the stereoacuity.

b. *Contrast sensitivity:* Contrast sensitivity again runs parallel to the outcome of vision in amblyopia therapy. However, in contrast to stereoacuity, contrast sensitivity shows better improvement after successful treatment in all types of amblyopia.

Motor Functions

It is best illustrated by 'hand–eye coordination'. After completion of amblyopia treatment, motor stability returns to normal and does not manifest any deficiency in later years.

Reading ability: Reading fluency and reading comprehension is a crucial development required for school age children. Reading was assessed monocularly in previously treated amblyopic patients using Gray Reading Test. The study showed amblyopic eyes were slower and less accurate in reading than normal eyes. Poorer visual acuity in amblyopic eye or slow processing by the brain may contribute to this result. Some studies have shown impaired 'binocular' reading impairment in amblyopia but this has not been confirmed.

The PEDIG Studies

Since no standardized protocol of amblyopia management existed, in 1997, the "Pediatric Eye Diseases Investigative Group" (PEDIG) was formed by the National Eye Institute, USA. The group is a collaborative network of around 60 centres involving more than 120 participating ophthalmologists. This is probably the largest authentic research group which had a broader investigative subject. Since the results of this group have opened new vistas in the management of amblyopia, it needs to be mentioned here. We will focus our attention on trial and inferences of studies related to amblyopia only.

1. *Best optical correction:* The general consensus reached was a trial of 'best optical correction' should be given in younger child with mild amblyopia. A time period of 6–8 weeks is reasonably good to achieve any result. The residual visual disparity, if remains, can be treated with methods of patching or atropine penalization.

2. *In number of PEDIG studies*, the regime of patching was studied regarding number of hours, severity of amblyopia, and age of patient. In young children aged 3 to 7 years with mild to moderate amblyopia, 2 hours patching had almost the same result, in terms of improvement of visual acuity, as compared to 6 hours of patching for 4 months. After 6 months of patching, the results were equal. Although 6 hours showed more rapid improvment in visual acuity. But many others have questioned the reliability of this regime regarding the compliance of patching. It is not ascertained how much time the child is actually putting the patch on the eye. It is commonly noticed that in any number of hours of patching advised, the actual time is usually less than advised. If so, then in so less time of patching, the results are always controversial. Nevertheless, it is a good idea to begin patching with 2 hours/day in mild amblyopia, and access the outcome after a month. If reasonable improvement in vision is occurring, then this regime may be continued.

   In severe amblyopias, 2 hours patching showed only partial improvement than 6 hours of patching. In older children, 7 years and above, net improvement in vision was much less satisfactory after 4 months of patching than patching of 6 hours or more.

3. *Atropine penalization:* One PEDIG study compared atropine 1% daily instillation with 6 hours of patching in a group of children aged 3–7 years with moderate amblyopia. Both groups showed almost equal improvement in vision after 6 months of treatment, i.e. 3 Snellen lines in patched group and 2.8 lines in the atropine group. This effect was similar in anisometropic and strabismic aetiologies.

This led to the recommendation by the group that patching of 6 hours/day had equal efficacy to atropine 1% use of daily dose. Thus either modality could be used for mild to moderate amblyopia. With this evidence-based result of atropine versus patching, an 'Amblyopia Treatment Index' was developed to assess the psychosocial impact on the child and family of amblyopia treatment. This 20-question test assesses quality-of-life issues with regard to various treatment modalities after 5 weeks of therapy. It has been internally validated with high reliability. The Amblyopia Treatment Index revealed that amblyopia treatment with atropine compared with patching was consistently better tolerated by the child and family with regard to the following factors, viz. adverse effect of treatment; better compliance; and social stigma. If fewer hours of patching was prescribed with patching 'only at home', away from school and friends, the social stigma scores were less negative. Daily atropine was also compared with 'once-a-week' atropine. In such a PEDIG study, after 4 months of treatment, the net improvement in vision was similar in both groups in mild to moderate amblyopia. The weekly dose showed better compliance and better tolerance. But the effectivity in severe amblyopias is questionable.

Cessation of Amblyopia Treatment

Risk of recurrence after one year of cessation of treatment varies from 6 to 60%, according to a PEDIG study. Recurrence was assessed as decrease of 2 lines from the final visual outcome.

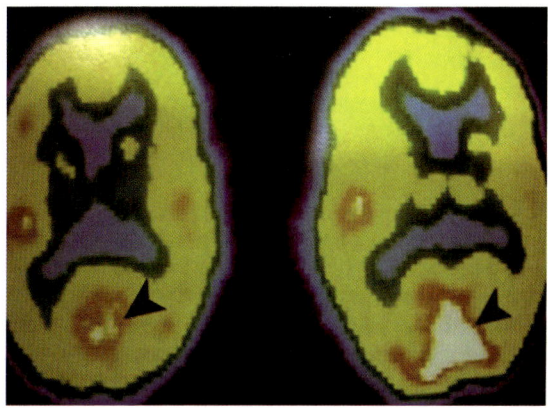

Fig. 7.4: Radio-isotope uptake study—left-normal person; right-amblyopic person showing deficient uptake

Recurrence rate was 25% in eyes which were patched and 24% which received atropine treatment. Recurrence rate was four times higher who abruptly stopped patching.

Other factors linked to recurrence are poor compliance, incorrect weaning schedule, patients who had faster improvement, large 'interocular vision disparity', incomplete vision improvement at the end of treatment, and previous history of recurrence.

Figure 7.4 compares a radio-isotope uptake in a non-functional visual cortex (right) to a functional cortex after treatment of amblyopia (left). The area is depicted by arrow.

Methodology of Ocular Examination in a Case of Amblyopia

It would be much easier, if the 'protocol' is explained taking an example.

A 6-year-old female presents to the eye clinic, having found defective vision in one eye at a routine school examination. She never complained of diminished vision or had any eye problems. Her parents also did not notice any abnormal visual behaviour or any complaints from the child. She was delivered normally and met satisfactorily all childhood milestones.

Ocular Examination

1. Visual acuity—by Snellen letters: OD 6/6; OS 6/24.
2. Extraocular motility—normal ductions and versions.
3. Ocular alignment—orthophoric at distance and near.
4. Stereotesting—positive with titmus fly; animals 1/3; wirt rings 0/9.
5. Pupillary reflex—no afferent pupillary defect in either eye.
6. Fields by confrontation method using toys—normal both eyes.
7. Cycloplegic refraction—OD +1.0/0.5 cyl 90; OS +3.0/+1.5 cyl 90
8. Other external eye examination—normal
9. Anterior segment examination—no abnormality detected.
10. Posterior segment examination—no abnormality detected.

Clinical Course

- The child was diagnosed as 'hyperopic anisometropia' with probable amblyopia, OS.
- She was advised glasses as per the following prescription: OD + 0.5 cyl 90 and OS +2.0/+1.5 cyl 90.
- It should be remembered that the accommodation acts according to the better eye; hence both eyes would accommodate 1 D. The remaining 2.0 D of the weak eye has to be compensated by external means. If this is not followed, then the presumed amblyopic eye would not accommodate and the vision would never be clear.
- The patient was reviewed after 6 weeks, as per the schedule. Her vision did not improve and the cycloplegic refraction had not changed. The child was initiated full-time occlusion, OD, and was recalled after one month.
- Her OS vision improved by 2 lines and at this return appointment, the mother reported that though the child accepted occlusion but did not put the patch for more than 5–6 hours. She resented patching in school and did not use while playing outdoors. Nevertheless, since even lesser number of hours of patching gave good results, the child and the parents were politely counselled about the beneficial

outcome of patching and were advised to continue patching in the same manner. After 4 months of regular patching—though less than the stipulated time—her vision improved to 6/6 part. Another one month of patching yielded the expected 6/6 visual acuity. The patching was then weaned as per the schedule described previously. This is a true story and one must now understand the mechanism of management of amblyopia.

Concept of Age in Amblyopia

1. *Age limit:* Traditionally, 7–8 years is the optimal age for best results of amblyopia therapy. In routine practice all over the world, 12 years of age is the upper limit when amblyopia therapy can be initiated. Beyond this age, the response has not been found satisfactory, although exceptions have been reported (this will be discussed later in this chapter). A PEDIG study in 2011, and later in UK, showed good results up to 13 years of age and even beyond! The meta-analysis of all recent studies concluded that maximum and aggressive treatment in older children should be non-hesitantly done, though the results may not be as good as in younger children. What has intrigued that even up to 17 or 18 years of age, some have shown dramatic response to treatment. The research group, however, was unable to identify the reasons for this response.

   In 1997, a report by Snowden and Stewart Brown, commissioned by the National Health Service, produced shock waves on their report of amblyopia therapy in older children. This prompted an explosion of research and renewed interest in the management of amblyopia.

   The later PEDIG studies and research sponsored by NHS in UK have to some extent constituted a protocol and paradigms for the management of amblyopia. At least we now have the go ahead to treat amblyopia even up to 18 years of age. There also have been isolated reports in the literature of recovery of vision even in adults! But most of these patients had undergone aborted treatment of amblyopia in childhood.

A recent report published entitled "Anisometropic Amblyopia—is the patient ever too old to treat", caused lot of amusement. This publication conducted a retrospective study of 19 patients ages 16 to 49 years. In addition to aggressive patching, an active vision therapy to develop monocular visual acuity and binocular function was also included. They concluded that these patients yielded long lasting' useful visual acuity and binocular function'. Though the exact visual acuity was not reported.

Ulffreda and colleagues in their book entitled *"Amblyopia: Basic and Clinical Approach"* stated that the end of period of susceptibility to treatment does not mark the end of period to initiate treatment. They also added that in many cases of amblyopia, some degree of 'residual plasticity' in brain remains present well into adulthood!

2. *Author's view:* Though there are isolated reports of treating amblyopia well beyond the teenage, but majority reports stated improvement in vision of not more than 2 or 3 lines on Snellen chart. Also most of these patients had undergone incomplete amblyopia treatment in some way in their early age. With all said and done, improvement in vision in later years still remains a mystery and results dubious; and initiation of amblyopia treatment at later ages should be undertaken with full counselling and clearly explaining the outcome of treatment.

Long-term follow-up of these patients pertaining to the maintenance of the improvement is also not mentioned in the literature.

Newer Modalities of Management

1. *Active stimulation:* A lot of interest has generated regarding 'active stimulation' for rapid and better recovery of vision. The following modalities are available:

   a. *'Near exercises'* are a set of modalities aimed at stimulating the visual system of the amblyopic eye. These include playing games on laptops; reading fine coloured prints; solving riddles; or playing with coloured blocks. The time devoted depends upon the severity of amblyopia, ranging from half hour to one hour. But their effectivity has shown equivocal results. The only positive aspect is that the patient and the parents are psychologically motivated for amblyopia treatment.

b. *CAM stimulator* (Cambridge) was an instrument to gently stimulate the foveal region. Initially, it generated a lot of interest and was intensively used for positive visual stimulation. But no added benefit was observed in randomized studies.

c. *Video games:* A study in Jerusalem, Israel, couple of years back, showed that watching 'violent video games' 2 hours a day along with patching for 2 hours/day only, had complete recovery of vision in moderate amblyopia. The recovery was faster than simply patching for 6 hours/day. This method of active stimulation showed promise and was recommended along with patching. The author uses this modality routnely for one hour but the patching schedule is not altered. This definitely expedites the improvement in visual acuity.

d. *Pleoptics:* This was a method devised by Bangerter, which consists of stimulation of fovea by flashes of controlled light or stimulation by Hadinger brushes. But this again did not yield any extra benefit in long-term studies as against simple patching with passive stimulation. This type of stimulation is not anymore practiced.

2. *Acupuncture:* Reports in 2011–12 by Dr Zhao from Ohio, USA have demonstrated promising results in mild to moderate amblyopia by 'acupuncture'. A controlled study on 80 children, aged 8–12, showed improvement of 2 to 3 lines in anisometropic amblyopia. The needles were inserted at 5 places around eyes and head, for 15 minutes five times a week for 16 weeks.

The work of Dr Zhao has been confirmed by Dr Zalman from University of Pennsylvania. The exact mechanism of action is not described. Probably these needles may be stimulating a particular area of neurons of the visual cortex.

3. *Neurotropic agents:* Mystry still surrounds that with all variables remaining constant in a group of patients, some

show drastic improvement while others remain resistant to treatment. The answer is as mysterious as the question! We have now come to understand that there is a definate regeneration or 'rejuvenation' of anatomic and functional architecture of the visual pathways and visual cortex during amblyopia therapy. We also understand that there is a catalytic role of many neurotransmitters and role of related neurotropic factors influencing the changes occurring in the recovery of the brain. The concept of 'plasticity' of the brain (visual cortex) is now undisputed. This plasticity or the ability of reformation extends far beyond the so-called critical period of visual recovery.

Therefore, to harness this capability of the visual cortex in particular, a tremendous amount of interest and research has generated in this field. Initially, dopamine and citicoline, known neurotransmitters in the brain, were tried as medical therapy for amblyopia, but did not yield any satisfactory result. Probably their mechanism of action does not affect the type of pathology in the visual cortex.

But the interest in this field continued. Attempts were made to enhance the activity of 'intrinsic' neurotropic agents. Jose Fernando et al. reported in Science Journal in 1998, that an anti-depressant agent 'fluoxetine' (Prozac) restores plasticity of the visual cortex.

Studies done in animals with long-term use of fluoxetine showed recovery of visual function in 'adult' amblyopic monkeys as tested electrophysiologically and behaviourly.

Another pathbreaking work by Maya Ventencourt reported in Journal of Physiology in 2009, showed a 'transcription factor Npas4' in the brain to be responsible for 'reactivating' the neuro-visual cortex in adult mice. Npas4 also showed to directly regulate the expression of ' brain-derived neurotropic factor (BDNF)', a molecule that has been clearly linked to multiple forms of synaptic plasticity and synaptic maturation.

There have been similar factors discovered in the brain that have been linked to synaptic development and maturation such as 'CREB', 'MEF2', OR 'NFAT' (West and Greenberg, 2011).

Drugs are being sought that can influence and increase the activity of these 'intrinsic neurotropic factors'. In this regard, research on serotonin is under way, and is showing good results.

Interactive Binocular Treatment (I-BiT)

This utilizes a computer-based programme, using commercially available 3-D shutter glasses. The treatment session consists of playing a computer game and watching a DVD through the I-BiT system. The system allows both eyes to see certain parts of image but only presents other parts of image to the amblyopic eye. Patients who undertook this study showed more than one line of improvement over and above the final result. The treatment was for 30 minutes every week for 6 weeks.

The rationale behind this binocular exercise is based on the recent assumptions that even in uniocular amblyopia, some types of binocular visual functions are also affected.

To summarize this issue, new vistas of treatment are emerging. Attempts and research is now directed to identify and develop certain drugs which have the potential to reactivate the plasticity of the visual cortex. As our knowledge into the intricacies of brain functioning widens, a time is not far enough when we will be able to 'restart' the dormant engine of the brain!

In a nutshell, following are the preferred practice recommendations for amblyopia treatment for all types of amblyopia

- For diagnosis and monitoring of amblyopia, measure the best corrected visual acuity with preferably LogMAR-based tests.
- Prescribe optical correction based on the cycloplegic refraction.
- Wear spectacles full time and monitor visual acuity after 6 weeks. If the visual acuity shows improvement, spectacles are continued, and patient reviewed every 6 weeks.
- If the visual acuity does not show any further improvement in the consecutive visit, then amblyopia therapy is initiated.
- If patching is preferred by the clinician, then the option of FTO versus PTO is to be decided.

- In mild to moderate amblyopias, in a young child, 2 to 4 hours of patching is done to begin with. If satisfactory response is not observed after 4 weeks, then the patching schedule is increased to 6 hours.
- In severe amblyopias and older children, full time patching for all waking hours (12 hours/day) is the treatment of choice.
- Atropine is usually not preferred as a primary mode of therapy. But certainly has a place in recurrences.
- If atropine penalization is chosen, then begin with twice weekly 1% atropine, and monitor vision every 4 weeks. If improvement remains same during two consecutive follow-up visits, then either the intensity of atropine is increased (daily schedule) or switch to another module. If patching has been the primary mode of therapy, then the time pattern is increased.
- Simultaneous active stimulation of fovea is introduced by video games or near exercises.
- In all instances, record stereoacuity at the beginning and during follow-up visits. A simple two pencil exercise promotes stereoacuity. Recording stereoacuity at each follow-up visits is a good added indicator of improvement of visual functions.
- The last limit of treatment is 6 months. With whatever method and most aggressive treatment, the maximum benefit is achieved by 6 months. Treatment beyond 6 months is usually not continued in its full force.
- After 6 months of therapy, which is the end point, the treatment is then gradually weaned.
- Follow-up is an integral part of management. Most cases of relapse are because of faulty weaning or failure of follow-up. Judicious follow-up is essential every 3 months for one year; then every 6 months for up to age 12 years.

Disability Associated with Amblyopia

Amblyopia is considered to be a childhood condition and it is mandatory that it is diagnosed and treated at this age only. Since these are the formative years of a child, both intellectually, psychologically and physically, clinicians need to know which life skills may be affected, apart from vision, if amblyopia goes untreated.

The most significant impact of amblyopia is that career choices become limited because of severe visual disability in one or both eyes. Moreover, loss of stereopsis and depth perception results in poor 'fine motor skills'. Good motor skills underlines many pre-school and school performances like handwriting and drawing. Bad hand writing and poor performances in sports, may affect a child's psychology, when they are often subjected to ridicule.

Psychosocial Development

The psychosocial implications of strabismus and amblyopia on an individual's quality of life have recently gained a lot of attention. Anecdotal references to the undesirable cosmetic appearance associated with an obvious strabismus have gained credence on an individual's self-esteem, interpersonal relationship and job opportunities.

A number of studies on this aspect reported that children with strabismus and amblyopia reported difficulty in self-image, interpersonal relations, school work and sports. The difficulties intensified in teenage and adult years, where patients demonstrated higher levels of stress. Amblyopic subjects were also found to experience more distress in areas of somatisation, obsession-compulsion, interpersonal sensitivity, anxiety and depression.

Amblyopia Management in Special Situations

There would be situations where a child being anisometropic, strabismic or both (mixed type) and having associated anomalies like cerebral palsy, delayed milestones, or other cerebral anomalies where correct assessment of visual acuity is difficult and, therefore, amblyopia management becomes a challenge and assessment of recovery of vision becomes difficult.

Nevertheless, perfect cycloplegic refraction followed by appropriate spectacle correction is the mainstay of initial treatment. Where ever surgery becomes mandatory in cases of pure strabismic amblyopia, it should be resorted to without delay, followed by amblyopia therapy.

Rule of the thumb is not always applied; wisdom and prudence should prevail. This is in context that amblyopia should be treated first, followed by surgical correction. Since the effect of amblyopia therapy cannot be assessed in such a child, perfect alignment of eyes is the first line of management. Also, as a reminder, it is advised that vision here can be tested by 'STYCAR' method, which has been devised by Sheridan and Gardiner particularly meant for handicapped children.

CONCLUSION

Although a tremendous amount of medical research has been conducted, one of the greatest challenges in medicine is there is a gap in applying research-based evidence to the process of making informed clinical decisions. Extrapolating this statement to amblyopia, there is no consensus on the most efficacious therapeutic modality. The intensity of treatment needed to maximize visual improvement is also widely debated. The diversity in opinions, therefore, emphasizes that optimum treatment for amblyopia is still unknown!

Part of uncertainty stems from the lack of 'standardization' in the management of amblyopia. Rules of the thumb do not always apply. Most of times, treatment has to be individualized as per the patient. There are confounding variables in the presentation of amblyopia, which makes it difficult to formulize a clear cut management. Experience of the clinician and compliance by the patient are the keys to a successful amblyopia management.

Newer modalities of treatment are fast emerging; role of neurotropic drugs seems to be very promising, but we will have to wait for the emergence of a exact drug to be helpful.

As of today, patching with its variants, accompanied by adjuvant therapy of active stimulation, remains the gold standard of treatment. In cases of all types of amblyopia, efforts to improve vision is the priority, as this is time bound, before embarking on surgical correction.

A good counselling to the child and parents is of paramount importance, as many times the treatment is taken casually, and its repercussions unknown to the family.

A thorough clinical examination, good counselling, an appropriate mode of therapy, and assessing the psychology of the child will go a long way for a fruitful management of amblyopia.

Cortical Visual Impairment

Cortical visual impairment (CVI) is a temporary or permanent vision impairment caused by a neurological problem affecting the posterior visual pathways or visual cortex, or both.

Typically, a child with CVI has a normal looking eye with a normal fundus, or has an eye condition that cannot account for the severity of vision loss. It is one of the most frequent causes of unexplained visual deficit in children.

In 2008, the American Printing House for the Blind brought together a large group of advisors and experts to provide guidance and clarity on issues related to CVI. The statements of such nationally drawn advisory group with incorporation of findings and conclusions of other clinicians form the basis of this chapter.

Cortical visual impairment is a complex subject, with wide array of symptoms and signs, often confusing to the patient as well as the clinician; and the intermixing of other cerebral disorders like cerebral palsy and delayed milestones. The problem is further compounded by rapid alteration in symptoms of the child, which adds to the complexity in arriving at an exact diagnosis. The disorder ranges from total cortical blindness to less severe visual impairment, to more lucid form of delayed milestones.

The severity of damage depends upon the type of insult, the time of insult, and the duration of injury.

Rapid development of brain takes place in early months of life, and any severe or prolonged damage may result in an irreparable, permanent damage. CVI is one of the most common infant neurological problem and 30 to 40% of children with visual dysfunction have CVI in some form or other.

A problem which all clinicians dealing with an assumed case of CVI faces is to distinguish between typical CVI and children having 'learning difficulties' or 'visual processing difficulties'.

A child with CVI would have the following specifications: (a) An examination that is completely normal, (b) a reliable history of an insult or damage to the brain, and (c) the presence of visual and behavioural symptoms that are collectively associated with CVI.

Some clinicians refer the term 'neurological visual impairment', which has three subsets, viz. cortical blindness, cortical visual impairment, and delayed visual maturation.

'Cortical blindness' is a term used when the vision is totally lost or the damage to the visual cortex is irreparable.

'Cortical visual impairment' is used in a condition where there has been partial loss of vision or recovery after the insult to the brain is not complete and a residual loss of vision has remained.

'Delayed visual maturation' is when maturation of visual pathways and/or visual cortex is delayed, but eventually the vision improves as the cerebral development proceeds. Initial examination would point towards CVI, but with time, the vision improves.

ETIOPATHOGENESIS

CVI can result from any insult or damage to the parts of brain concerned with vision. For better understanding, CVI may be divided into (1) congenital, and (2) acquired. Congenital causes include decreased blood supply to the brain, birth asphyxia/ hypoxia, brain malformations, cerebral infections, septicaemia, hydrocephalus, meningitis, seizures, metabolic diseases, drug toxicity, birth trauma, and other neurological congenital affections. The most common cause of CVI is cerebral ischaemia (oxygen deprivation) to the visual cortex, which may be transient or prolonged.

Secondary reasons include vascular lesions of visual cortex, side effect of antiepileptic drugs, Creutzfeldt-Jacob disease, encephalitis/meningitis, head trauma, hyperaminuria, brain malformations, seizures, etc.

Studies done by different clinicians on aetiology, recovery of vision, and type of affliction showed most cases resulting from birth asphyxia or head trauma.

Poor visual outcome occurred in patients with severe birth hypoxia, status epilepticus, intracranial haemorrhage, cerebral thrombosis, and head injury. Good visual recovery occurred in children with transient hypoxia or hypotensive episodes of short duration or recovery after brain surgery for infantile tumours. Recovery period in these cases was from 6 weeks to 6 months.

PATHOLOGY

Insult of any sort, as listed in aetiology, can result in damage to the visual functions, but differs prognostically to the area affected. Pathology in the geniculate or post-geniculate optic radiations have variable vision loss, but injury to the visual and adjacent cortex usually leads to severe and permanent visual loss.

Literature reports some cases of transient total loss of vision following mild, trivial head injury to the occipital cortex. A type of syndrome has been observed where children with seemingly trivial blunt head trauma had complete visual loss ranging from a few minutes to a few hours. No neurological deficit was observed and no abnormality was noticed in CT/ MRI. Vision totally recovered after a few minutes to a few hours and no long-term deficit was noted.

Characteristics of CVI

Visual characteristics associated with CVI are:
1. Distinct colour preferences
2. Variable vision loss
3. Difficulty in responding to complex visual stimuli
4. Delayed visual response

5. Difficulty in visualizing new surroundings and objects
6. Better vision in lighted areas
7. Preference for viewing near objects
8. Better vision for moving objects than static objects (Riddoch syndrome)
9. Denial of vision loss (Anton-Babinski phenomenon)
10. Visual hallucinations
11. Macular sparing in some cases
12. Difficulty in recognizing known faces
13. Getting lost at new surroundings
14. Spatial difficulties, i.e. missing steps, depth perception problems.

CLINICAL FEATURES

CVI has a wide range of symptoms and each child may have combination of different signs and symptoms. The most significant part of CVI concerning the clinician is the vision of the child.

CVI exhibits variable vision. The acuity may fluctuate many times in a day or even every a few minutes, especially when the child is tired. Patients suffering from this affliction should be prepared for such fluctuations and must carry some support such as a walking-cane when outdoors.

One eye may perform significantly worse than the other and depth perception is very limited.

The field of vision may be restricted, sometimes only tubular vision may remain. One of classical symptoms is that more often the vision is centred at some other point; so it becomes difficult to comprehend what the patient is actually looking at!

Though the child's vision may not be clear, but he/she is able to 'detect and track' movement. Motion is handled by area V5 of visual cortex (extra-striate area) which may have escaped the damage. Sometimes a moving object is seen better than a stationary one; while at other times a person can sense movement but cannot recognize what is moving. However, fast motion is usually deficient and a fast moving object simply 'disappears'. Objects with highly reflective properties can be better seen as they simulate movement! But too many objects moving together can cause confusion and the brain then ignores them.

Some objects may be better seen than others; e.g. faces or facial expressions may be difficult to recognize but may identify written material.

Colour and contrast is another area variably affected in CVI. The brain's colour processing system is distributed in such a way that it escapes damage to quite an extent, unless a very large area is damaged.

So colour perception may be preserved in most cases; yellow and red are easier to recognize, as long as contrast is good.

Persons with CVI strongly prefer 'simplified' viewing. For example, the written text should not be extensive, a few lines at a time. The letters should be large and the child may bring it closer for magnification. Good illumination further facilitates the reading.

In viewing an array of objects, a CVI patient prefers to view one or two objects at a time. Familiar objects are preferred over unfamiliar objects; strong contrast or bright illumination is desirable.

Similarly, children with CVI avoid crowded atmosphere or crowded rooms, as their limited visual function is more dependent on simple or single objects! This avoidance of 'visual cluster' is one of the characteristic signs of CVI.

Visual processing of the retinal image takes a lot of effort in these patients. They have to make a choice in viewing multiple objects as which one to be preferred. The visual cortex has to make a strenuous effort to arrive at a conclusion. Also the brain cannot maintain fixation for long at a particular object. For same reasons, the person cannot keep eye contact for long and shifts eye contact from one person to another, sometimes creating an embarrassing situation.

It is also difficult for some to look at a particular object and then reach for it! These two tasks are performed by two different areas of brain and it depends which one is more severely affected.

Approximately, one-third of children with CVI have photophobia. It also takes longer to adjust to changes to illumination and flashes of light can be painful. On the contrary, in some cases, there is a desire to gaze compulsively at light sources.

Children with CVI assume what they see is the real one; but on closer look, the object may turn out to be a different in reality. Thus, they may suffer from illusions and perceive a picture differently than a normal person would see.

In a nutshell, it is to be understood that a child with CVI has varied and mixture of signs and symptoms and not all classical characteristics are present in each case. It is, therefore, difficult as to what exact therapy should be instituted as the symptoms may contradict a standard therapy.

Because children with CVI have additional disabilities, it is sometimes difficult to measure the visual acuity. Wherever possible, visual acuity should be carefully recorded using the age-specific tests. Electrophysiological tests, like VEP, can be used where direct vision assessment is inconclusive.

A recent study tries to clarify 'pure CVI' from other associated problems owing to damage to other areas of brain. Children with perceptual and cognitive dysfunction may have cerebral processing problems that do not represent 'visual dysfunction'. CVI, on the other hand, is a cortical disorder that conforms to a 'unique set of visual and behavioural symptoms'. In a nutshell, consensus has emerged that CVI should be considered a sub-set of a broadly defined term 'cerebral visual impairment'. Thus, a patient of with CVI may also have cognitive disorder, cerebral palsy, hearing loss, seizures, etc. In addition to impaired vision, children who are diagnosed with CVI also demonstrate the phenotype characteristics of CVI. As with ocular pathology, the severity of CVI should be considered across a spectrum—ranging from mild, moderate to severe. The visual acuity, other visual conditions and other co-morbid cerebral conditions can vary with individuals. In addition, some variations in symptoms occur depending on fluctuations in environment, health, treatment and effect of rehabilitation.

Fortunately, most children show improvement in vision with time; but many continue to show typical CVI characteristics throughout life.

Vision Assessment in CVI

Many a times, it is difficult to assess the exact visual acuity in these children; following are some pearls to help assess vision:

1. Present large, high contrast, lighted objects.
2. Presentation of material from different angles.
3. Material to be presented as single objects; avoid clustering.
4. Material with ample illumination; i.e. lighted toys against dim background illumination.
5. 'Observe and assess', to gain some visual information, when no scientific tools work.
6. Child should be well fed, not sleepy and in ambient environment.

Other ancillary modes of examination are: (a) Visually evoked potential (VEP), (b) electroencephalography, (c) magnetic resonance imaging (MRI).

DIAGNOSIS

Diagnosis of CVI is difficult. Previously, it was thought that the child is faking; but newer techniques of diagnosis, like MRI and VEP, and electrical responses of retina (ERG), have helped in diagnosis.

A patient with typical CVI has none or severely reduced vision, but the pupillary reactions are intact. The fundus is normal and the eye as a whole shows no defects. Persons with CVI may not be able to distinguish an object but may be able to reveal its colour or its general shape. This indicates that the deficit is not ocular and that the visual cortex is not able to process and interpret the visual stimuli from the eyes. Sensitive tools of diagnosis like MRI, VEP, characteristic visual responses, and a careful history, often clinches the diagnosis.

TREATMENT AND PROGNOSIS

In cases of acquired CVI, the mainstay of treatment is correct, early diagnosis and prompt intervention. As with all cerebral tissues, neurological development is rapid in early years of life and thus acquired neurological disorders, if promptly and properly treated, rarely give rise to a permanent cortical visual blindness. They usually slip into 'cortical visual 'impairment'.

Similarly, congenital or perinatal insults, like eclampsia or transient hypoxia during birth or mild birth head trauma, do not have a lasting effect on vision and the recovery is prognostically good.

Children having suffered from drug toxicity, the loss is usually reversible and a complete recovery of vision is predictable.

Recent research on 'relearning of complex visual motion' following damage to V1 area of cortex has offered potential promise of treatment and result. These treatments focus on 'retraining and retuning' of certain intact pathways to the visual cortex which are more or less preserved. This sort of 'relearning exercise' may provide a good work around for persons with acquired cortical injury in order to make better sense of the visual environment.

In past two decades, several theoretical and remedial perspectives have emerged that are related to classification models of CVI so that specific management can be accorded depending upon the severity of CVI and intervention strategies based on behavioural characteristics.

Children suffering from congenital malformations or disorders in brain should be promptly addressed by surgery and/or other means, so that permanent damage is prevented.

Those who have suffered irreparable damage and present characteristic features of CVI, should be provided special training and vocational programs for rehabilitation. They would come in the category of 'severely visually impaired' and the relevant management should be instituted.

Accommodative Anomalies in Children

INTRODUCTION

Accommodation is one of the greatest virtues we use to see clearly and comfortably. There are quite a few of visual problems which arise while using the eyes for near work, where accommodation comes into effect; but unfortunately, this aspect has been least studied and disregarded. Ocular asthenopia and host of related problems arising on near work have never been scientifically attributed to anomalies in accommodation. More so, such problems have never been even thought to arise in children—as their accommodation is assumed to be great and flawless. This is a big misbelief which we have nurtured all along. Though this concept has been studied for many years and we have now a clear understanding of the accommodative mechanism, but it is rarely clinically applied in practice. Symptoms on near work like headaches, asthenopia, watering, blurring, redness, lack of concentration, etc. occur frequently in children, and every test is done from refraction to ocular motility, to find the cause, except accommodative tests.

But it may come as a surprise that accommodation is not as efficient in children as expected. Number of studies have now clearly stated that in case of above symptoms, a thorough accommodative tests should also be carried out. Subjective symptoms usually emerge around 6–7 years of age when children start getting extensively involved in near work, and there is a clear relationship between accommodative parameters and these symptoms. Because accommodative dysfunctions may result in varied asthenopic symptoms, it is of utmost importance to identify this dysfunction to prevent unnecessary visual problems. Therefore, clear standards for diagnosing an accommodative dysfunction need to be further refined. Studies have shown that accommodative training, in cases of dysfunction, is an effective method in alleviating the symptoms.

BASICS OF ACCOMMODATION

1. Anatomically, three parts in the eye are involved in the accommodative process, i.e. (a) ciliary muscles—circular and meridional, (b) the zonules, and (c) the crystalline lens.

   By far, most of attention has been through a single window, the crystalline lens, in the accommodative mechanism; very little focus has been given to the muscles which are the primary partner in this process. It is now becoming evidently clear that accommodative anomalies, especially in children, are primarily situated in the muscles.

2. The characteristics of effective 'accommodative stimuli', are the first step in our understanding of accommodative system. There are a number of 'different' accommodative stimuli which stimulate accommodation to varying degrees. These are:

   - Blur of the object
   - Proximity of the target
   - Changing target size
   - Chromatic aberration
   - Convergence of eyes
   - Spatial frequency

These are all different stimuli to accommodation with 'blur' of object having the greatest impact as an stimuli, though independent of visual acuity.

An important implication is the completely different character of these stimuli, which can act together as well as independently.

Amplitude of Accommodation

The ability to focus a visual target at varying distances is known as accommodation, and is present to some extent from birth, but improves rapidly by first 6 months of life. It is believed that a small child is able to focus from infinity down to very close to the eyes because of high level of accommodation. However, it is to be noted that accommodation and convergence are not automatically linked from the start. The amount of accommodation, in diopters, needed to clearly focus an object from infinity to the nearest point possible, is the 'amplitude of accommodation'.

The accommodative function is normally expressed by describing the accommodative amplitude and its dioptric value. However, the accommodative function is more complicated than that. The accommodative system is complex, and comprises of not only the amplitude but number of other functions; any of them can be underdeveloped and can give rise to ocular symptoms. Therefore, the object of this chapter is to apprise the reader of various facets of accommodative system and the implications it has on the subjective symptoms in a child.

Different Facets of Accommodation

1. Amplitude of accommodation
2. Tonic accommodation
3. Lag of accommodation
4. Convergence accommodation
5. Accommodative facility
6. Relative accommodation.

These facets differ greatly from each other with regard to function. They require different methods of measurement and are not explained by the same dioptric value. There is no method in use that describes the complete accommodative function, nor we use the same measuring system for different dioptric results. Furthermore, dysfunction of each envisages different set of symptoms.

Let us review each of these facets.

1. *Amplitude of accommodation:* As already stated, it is the total accommodative power of the eye and is expressed in dioptric equivalent and is reciprocal to the distance of the object from the eye. As age advances, the power of accommodation deteriorates, and the ability to see clearly at near diminishes. As a matter of fact, this ability or facet of accommodation is most relevant to the clinician and thus, is the only one tested clinically in routine practice.

   Amplitude tests:

   a. *Donders push-up method:* This uses the RAF ruler (also known as Prince ruler). In this, a ruler about 50 cm in length has markings on one side in cm and other side in dioptres. A sliding box is mounted on the ruler in which letter lines conforming to Snellen's optotype size to be read from near. The subject holds the ruler with one end mounted on nose and holds the other end with the hand. A +3.0 D lens is placed in front of eyes to pull up the range of accommodation to 35 cm. The reading card or box is moved away till the print blurs and pulled up near till the print blurs again. The difference between the two readings gives the amplitude of accommodation.

   b. *Sheard's method:* Here, minus lenses are added at far distance target, monocularly or binocularly, until blur at distance occurs. The power of lenses used gives the amplitude.

2. *Tonic accommodation:* Tonic accommodation (TA) or dark accommodation (DA) is a passive state of accommodation in the absence of any stimulus. This occurs when the eye is in complete darkness or when it is looking at a bright empty field. Basically, it is the inherent tone of the ciliary muscles when the eye is at rest. Ironically, the resting 'tone' varies in different situations or differs in refractive errors.

   This tonic state of accommodation or the 'resting state tone' of the ciliary muscles can be unearthed only after total cycloplegia. Another way of measuring is by using an objective 'infrared optometer.'

3. *Lag of accommodation:* The amount by which the accommodative response of the eye is less than the diopteric stimulus to accommodation is defined as the 'accommodative lag'. Clinical measurement of accommodative lag at near is typically done by dynamic retinoscopy. This is an objective method in which the patient views a near point target, while the examiner uses lenses to neutralize the fundal glow movement.

4. *Convergence accommodation:* Convergence accommodation is normally described by the ratio between convergence accommodation and convergence, or the CA/C ratio.

   The ratio is the measure of the effect of change in convergence on accommodation.

   It is expressed as the change in accommodation (dioptre) for each change in convergence in prism dioptre.

5. *Accommodative facility:* 'Accommodative facility' is the ability to rapidly change the power of the crystalline lens to various focus distances while maintaining a requisite angle of convergence (binocularly) or eliminating the influence of convergence (monocularly). This ability is important while changing the fixation from near to distance and back again.

   Clinically, accommodative facility can be measured using lenses that stimulate accommodation (minus lenses) or inhibit accommodation (plus lenses). Any combination can be used for evaluation, but experience has shown that plus-minus 2D is a reasonable choice. The procedure uses plus-minus 2D lens pair mounted on a 'flipper frame'. A flipper is a frame on which two plus and two minus lenses are mounted.

   The subject focuses through one pair of lenses at an object at fixed distance (say 40 cm). When the object is clearly focused, a 'flip' of the frame is quickly performed to bring the other pair in front of eyes, and the person focuses through them. This is then again repeated; and the number of cycles completed in one minute is noted as the 'accommodative facility' in 'cycles/min' (cpm).

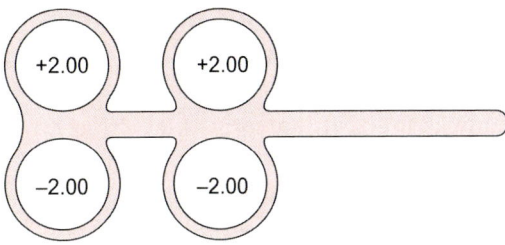

Fig. 9.1: Flipper test

Normative data on children have been collected by number of researchers. The results of the Flipper test in children aged 6–12 years were 5.0 + –2.5 cpm, in one study and 4.0 + –2.5 cpm in another study.

The cutoff parameter for reduced facility to show symptoms is less than 3 cpm.

The facility testing is important and has bearing on the symptoms where children complain in difficulty in focusing on the board and then reading/writing at near (Fig. 9.1).

6. *Relative accommodation:* The total amount of accommodation, which can be exerted while the convergence remaining fixed, is called the 'relative accommodation'. This can be either 'positive relative accommodation (PRA) or 'negative relative accommodation' (NRA).

PRA is the amount of accommodation in excess of the accommodation needed for convergence and NRA is the amount of accommodation less than needed for convergence. In other words, the least amount of accommodation or maximum relaxation of accommodation with which one can see clearly at a fixed distance is the NRA and the maximum accommodation used over and above the need at a fixed distance is called PRA. To assess this flexibility, a simple test is used. With a vergence stimulus fixed at 40 cm, positive lenses with 0.25 D increment are put in front of both eyes and the first sign of blur is noted. The amount of plus lenses used will give the value of NRA. Similarly, now minus lenses are used with increasing power in 0.25 D steps, binocularly, till the first sign of blur is noted. The increased amount stimulus at this point is the PRA.

Tests for PRA and NRA are very helpful in determining accommodative dysfunctions in children. A low NRA reveals accommodative spasticity; while a low PRA suggests that the focusing mechanism may be prone to tiring after concentrated near work.

It would be not out of place to discuss about the **accommodative convergence/accommodation ratio** (AC/A ratio); as it is linked with accommodation. Due to the near vision reflex complex, a certain amount of convergence is expected when accommodation is in force. The relation between the dioptric change in accommodation and the prismatic change in convergence is called the AC/A ratio. In simple terms, the AC/A ratio describes how much convergence is activated by an accommodative change of 1 D. Normally, convergence of 3–5 PD occurs when 1 D of accommodation is exerted. An AC/A of 10 or more is termed as high ratio while an AC/A ratio of less than 3 is termed as low.

Practical Dysfunctions

The accommodative system at young age is quite flexible and resistant to fatigue. However, in clinical practice, accommodative dysfunction can occur in children and young people. Often children and teenagers complain of certain symptoms which appear when doing near work. The refractive system is usually emmetrope or slightly ametropic, but that is not always in relation to the complaints. Unfortunately, there does not exist, as mentioned earlier, no simple, single standard procedure, which might include all facets of accommodative dysfunction. Because of this reason and because we do not have any clear cut method of treating accommodative problems, the accommodative system is not routinely examined. But it is of great importance to identify any accommodative dysfunction, if any complaints exist, so that unnecessary near vision problems may be prevented. It is also important to identify any accommodative dysfunction or deficiency in school-going children, because this has a bearing on the performance of children in school. Because the focusing system of eyes has contribution in the learning process, any accommodative deficiency can make it unnecessarily difficult for the child to read and write and develop in studies. If the child's accommodative deficiencies are not resolved, he/she may develop dislike in near work and develop lack of interest in studies. Therefore, we need to find a simple and easy-to-use method that identifies an accommodative dysfunction.

It is difficult to group together accommodative dysfunctions, as the boundaries are often unclear. However, clinically it is useful to separate anomalies of accommodation into five distinct 'syndrome categories.'

1. Insufficiency of accommodation
2. Infacility of accommodation
3. Fatigue of accommodation
4. Spasm of accommodation
5. Paresis of accommodation

These five syndromes constitute different accommodative disorders, having slightly different sysmptoms, having different impact on accommodative function.

A brief description of each would be helpful in identifying and treating the disorders.

An important aspect is that symptoms related to accommodative dysfunction must be clearly recognized and understood. Most of times, the clinician concentrates only on the refractive anomalies, and attributes all symptoms to the refractive problem. It should be remembered that all symptoms need not be due to refractive error; time should be devoted to enquire about various symptoms especially arising from near work and tests should be employed to determine the type of accommodative anomaly.

Understanding the symptoms is of paramount importance in recognizing any accommodative anomaly.

Asthenopia is a cardinal symptom which stands out prominently in accommodative deficiencies. 'Asthenopia' is a term used to describe eye strain or symptoms arising from use of eyes for near work.

Though asthenopia is used loosely to describe all types of symptom but scientifically explaining, it means purely eye strain and comprises of red eyes, frequent rubbing and irritation of eyes, and disinterest in doing near work after a certain time. Other symptoms arising of accommodative strain are headaches, diplopia, blurring, vertigo, and drowsiness.

As asthenopia is the flag bearer of any ocular morbidity, it would not be out of place to illustrate the reasons of asthenopia. Asthenopia, *per se*, can occur in the following conditions:

1. Accommodative insufficiency
2. Accommodative infacility
3. Accommodative fatigue
4. Accommodative spasm
5. Dyslexia
6. Hysteria
7. Ocular inflammations
8. Phorias—ocular motility disorders
9. Latent nystagmus
10. Anisekonia
11. Refractive errors: Astigmatim; hyperopia; anisometropia
12. Accommodative paresis.

It thus becomes mandatory to recognize these conditions by exclusion and look for the accommodative reasons carefully.

Since this chapter is dedicated to accommodative problems, let us briefly discuss the five syndromes which occur clinically.

1. *Insufficiency of accommodation:* It is a condition in which the amplitude of accommodation is chronically below the lower limits of expected amplitude of accommodation for the person's age. Classically, insufficiency of accommodation is a physiological phenomenon of advancing age and very rare in children. But studies have shown that this problem is not too uncommon in children. In one study in children aged 10–15 years, with low accommodative amplitude, had severe complaints of asthenopia, headaches, diplopia and difficulty in reading. Therefore, the clinical recognition of accommodative insufficiency is important in preventing unwanted frustration in school-going children. The clinician

should keep his mind open where such accommodative insufficiency is suspected, especially in circumstances of certain syndromes or the child is on drugs for psychological disorders.

2. *Infacility of accommodation:* As previously discussed, this is a condition in which a rapid change of accommodation from far to near and *vice-versa* is failing and raises symptoms of asthenopia. It differs from insufficiency in that clear vision is eventually achieved, albeit after some time. If changing fixation from distance to near takes more than one second, an abnormal condition is likely to be present. Children who need to change fixation rapidly from distance to near, as is commonly done in school in viewing blackboard and then writing at near, start complaining of ocular pain or headaches after long hours in school.

3. *Fatigue of accommodation:* Fatigue of accommodation is described as the inability of ciliary muscle to maintain contraction while viewing a near target with a resulting blurring of the object and shift of accommodation towards far point. Normally, in young children, the amplitude is so much in reserve that this condition is rare. If in a child there is doubt of such a situation, then a thorough cycloplegic refraction is warranted to weed out hyperopia or astigmatism. Still, the reading habits and light source should also be enquired into.

4. *Spasm of accommodation:* Spasm of accommodation is a constant or intermittent involuntary and inappropriate ciliary contraction. It may be unilateral or bilateral. Symptoms include distance and/or near blur, visual distortion, constant browache or headaches, and sometimes diplopia. Also a dynamic retinoscopy shows no change.

5. *Paresis of accommodation:* Paresis of accommodation could be partial or complete.

The most common cause of paresis is use of cycloplegic drops whether deliberate or inadvertent. It is to be understood that the use of cycloplegic drops used for refraction have a duration of effect; but it may not be surprising, if the effect continues well beyond the stipulated time frame. In every case of suspected cycloplegic used, whether at your clinic or elsewhere, the type and date of refraction must be enquired.

Accommodative paresis can also be functional, owing to weakness or fatigue of ciliary muscles.

Near work performance can also be hampered due to certain accommodative syndromes, neurological disorders, use of certain sedatives, anticholinergic drugs, antipsychotic drugs, hysteria, etc. The 'accommodative facility' can be inherently deficient despite the amplitude being normal; thus a thorough tests of various facets of accommodation should be done to arrive at a correct diagnosis of accommodative problem.

ACCOMMODATIVE THERAPY

Accommodative dysfunctions is not an uncommon visual anomaly in children and the symptoms typically occur during near work. Out of the dysfunctions mentioned above, accommodative 'insufficiency' and accommodative 'infacility' are the most common dysfunctions encountered in children. After ruling out neurological, pharmaceutical and general health issues, the standard treatment of accommodative dysfunction is generally orthoptic exercises or addition of plus lens for near.

In cases of accommodative insufficiency, what is needed is a proper distance correction with an addition of appropriate plus lenses for near. Orthoptic exercises to strengthen vergence or accommodation by 'push-up' technique should also be employed.

A plus lens add is recommended in cases of excessive 'lag of accommodation', 'very low PRA', or 'fatigue of accommo-dation'. The prescription can be either in form of normal reading glasses or bifocals.

Orthoptic exercise is a sequence of activities individually prescribed and monitored by the clinician to develop efficient visual skills and processing. 'Flipper' method is an extremely efficient method aimed at developing accommodative efficiency and 'push-up' exercise to strengthen vergence and accommo-dation. Use of synoptophore is a time tested machine for orthoptic exercises, but the patient's regular attendance is doubtful; even home-based exercises have proved to be equally effective and should be relied upon.

There is a scientific and clinical evidence to support the efficiency of using facility therapy techniques to strengthen or improve accommodative functions.

CONCLUSION

The knowledge of how the neuronal accommodative system functions is still limited. The general consensus that young children or teenagers, with strong accommodative amplitudes are immune to accommodative anomalies, is misleading. Wayback in 1912, Duane stated that the amplitude of accommodation is quite high in young children. Furthermore, Berens and Sells (1944) pointed out that accommodation in young children is extremely flexible and resistant to fatigue. Though this old data is still what we normally believe, the ocular accommodation in children is not as sufficient or efficient as we expect. There is no simple standard procedure which includes all accommodative facets for examination. The accommodative system is, therefore, not routinely examined because of lack of such method and more so because of the concept that there cannot be any fallacy of accommodation in children. Young school children may have an insufficient accommodative ability that causes subjective symptoms when reading. Excluding all pathological or pharmaceutical entities, a 'general weakness' in a child is enough to cause near work dysfunctions. Therefore, it is prudent and mandatory to look for these anomalies and take seriously any complaints arising out of near work in children.

A proper cycloplegic refraction is primary to all complaints, whether or not the visual acuity is normal. After a correct lens prescription, if the complaints persist, then a thorough accommodative tests should be performed. Accommodative spasm is not infrequent in an uncorrected hyperope, specially if the person is involved in excessive, long near work—as in computer work. The ordeal of 'computer vision syndrome' is now well documented. But we rarely go into the tests for accommodative anomalies arising in this syndrome.

With all said and done, near work complaints and problems are on the increase in children, courtesy computers and mobile game gadgets, and as a vigilant clinician it is imperative that we take the near vision complaints of children seriously and make a conscience effort to look for accommodative anomalies.

Learning Disorders

Learning disabilities or disorders are an umbrella term for a wide variety of learning problems. A learning disorder is not a deficiency of intelligence, or motivation or vision.

Children with learning disabilities are also not lazy or dumb. The reason why this chapter is included in this book is two-fold. One, a large number of children who read and write incorrectly are repeatedly subjected to eye examinations. Having found no refractive error or any ocular defect on a judicious eye testing on number of occasions, are never satisfied that their ward does 'not' have an eye disorder. Secondly, every ophthalmologist must be aware of this problem and should have a vivid understanding what the child is actually suffering from. Once this is ascertained, the parents can be guided and counselled accordingly.

Simply put, children and teenagers with learning disorders see, write, and understand differently. This leads to trouble in identifying letters and words, difficulty in learning new information and skills, and putting them to use. The most common types of learning disabilities involve problems with reading, writing, calculations, reasoning, listening, and speaking. These disabilities manifest differently and in varying degrees in symptoms from one child to another. Some children struggle with reading and spelling, while others love reading but confuse in writing or calculations. Still others have difficulty in communicating or understanding what others are saying.

A brief description of these disorders deserves mention in this chapter. Dyslexia, the most common and most closely associated with vision, needs detail description.

DYSLEXIA

Definition

Dyslexia is a specific reading disorder due to a defect in the brain's processing of graphic symbols. It is a learning disability that alters the way the brain processes written material. It is typically characterized by difficulties in word recognition, spelling and decoding. People with dyslexia have problems with reading comprehension. There is also associated problems in speaking, writing and understanding spoken language.

It is a complex disorder and in wild cases, it becomes difficult to arrive at a precise diagnosis. It is to be clearly understood that dyslexia is a neurological problem, and not linked to poor vision, poor learning or poor upbringing.

Clinical Features

According to most studies, dyslexia is the most common learning disability. Almost 15–20% of general population have some of the symptoms of dyslexia. Dyslexia varies from person-to-person in severity and varying in symptoms. It includes slow or inaccurate reading, poor spelling, poor writing, or mixing up similar words. These characteristics vary in severity. Many a times, the child is often scolded for not paying attention or concentrating. At other times, the slow reading may be so annoying that the child is often labelled as mentally retarded or having poor milestones. It is assumed that the milestones of the child are delayed and the parents are advised good diet for the child and to wait patiently. But this is not so. Delay in instituting timely treatment not only prolongs the disorder but leaves the child in mental agony as he/she is often rebuked and ridiculed.

Boys are 2–3 times more affected than girls. All ethnic groups are equally affected and the disorder is prevalent worldwide. Genetic predisposition is assumed as a major causative factor.

The following are the most common signs and symptoms associated with dyslexia:

1. *Learning to read:* The child in spite of having normal intelligence and receiving proper education has difficulty in learning to read.

2. *Milestones:* In many cases, the development of milestones is delayed. Central milestones like crawling, walking, talking, playing games are delayed.

3. *Speech:* Apart from being slow to learn to speak, the child constantly mispronounces the words, finds rhyming difficult, and does not appear to distinguish between different word sounds.

4. *Slow learner:* At school, a child takes much longer than other children to learn the letters of alphabet and how they are pronounced. Even on repeated training, the child pronounces certain letters incorrectly. There may also be problem in remembering days of a week, months of the year, colours, etc.

5. *Reversal of letters:* One of the prominent features of dyslexia is reversal of letter or number. The person, confuses between 'b' and 'd', or 'q' and 'p', 'was' and 'saw', etc. Similarly, 'left' and 'right' get mixed off without realizing.

6. *Coordination:* A child may seem clumsier than his compatriots. Catching a ball may look clumsy to the on-lookers.

7. *Spelling:* Learning a spelling and then reproducing it may seem difficult in some children. He may learn a spelling today and may forget it the next day. More than that, the child may spell the same word differently on the same page. All this may seem that child is not seeing properly and would become eligible for ophthalmic examination.

8. *Phonology problems:* Phonology refers to the speech sounds in a language. Suppose a word has number of syllables, then the child may not be able to pronounce all of them. For example, in the word 'unfortunately', a person with

dyslexia may be able to process the sounds 'un' and 'tely', but not be able to process the ones in between.

9. *Concentration problems:* A child with dyslexia may not be able to concentrate too long, as compared to other children. They may get distracted or complain of exhaustion resulting in headaches or eye aches. This is another reason for their referral to an ophthalmologist. This must be distinguished from ADD (attention deficit disorder), though many of dyslexia patients manifest ADD and ADHD.

10. *Sequencing ideas:* When a persons with dyslexia narrates a sequence of ideas, he may seem illogical or irrelevant at many times.

11. *Immunological disorders:* Dyslexia persons are more prone to immunological problems like hay fever, asthma, eczema, etc.

Etiopathogenesis of Dyslexia

Genetics: Since dyslexia is seen to run in families, a genetic cause has been hypothesized. Recent studies have shown that defects in genome DCDC2 and KIAAO319 genes are responsible for some traits of dyslexia. But the genetic predisposition is more complex with more number of genes involved in dyslexia.

The inheritance traits appear to affect parts of the brain concerned with language comprehension, interfering with the ability to convert letters and words into speech.

Acquired dyslexia: Apart from being a congenital condition, a small number of patients manifesting dyslexic signs and symptoms are acquired in nature. The most common conditions being stroke, head injuries, vascular insufficiency to the brain, etc.

Phonological processing: People with dyslexia find reading and writing difficult because of 'phonological processing impairment'. Humans have the ability to understand spoken language; something that the brain acquires easily and naturally from a very early age. This natural ability to acquire and understand language, explains the reason why, when we listen to verbal communication, we do not consciously register that the words are made of 'phonemes'; we only hear the word itself. Phonemes are the small unit of sound that words are made of.

For example, in a word 'elephant', we do not break it into 'ele-pha-nt' and again assemble it. This happens when we are learning to hear and make sense of it. But when we are learning to read and write, we first learn about the letters which make up the word, then identifying the phonemes, putting it together to make a complete word. This is called 'phonological processing'. Persons with dyslexia have problems with phonological processing and, therefore, have difficulty in writing and pronouncing the word properly.

Diagnosing Dyslexia

Dyslexia is a complex problem. Until it is not correctly diagnosed, it is assumed that the child has vision problem. Also, the diversity and variation in severity of symptoms makes it go unnoticed many a times.

There are certain tests to diagnose dyslexia, but the tests and how they should be performed will vary depending on the age of the patient and the type of problem they have. When testing children, the examination will focus on phonological processing, how well the child expresses himself or herself, and their ability to make 'sound-symbol' associations.

Ideally a test should cover the following points:
1. Background information
2. Intelligence
3. Language skills
4. Word recognition
5. Phonological processing
6. Reading fluency skills
7. Vocabulary knowledge
8. Family history and milestones.

In assessing or diagnosing dyslexia, the examiner must rule out certain conditions which may show similar symptoms like vision problems, hearing defects, lack of education, social and economic problems. Vision problems are perhaps the most significant and most confusing in differentiating dyslexia. It is mandatory that all children with problems in reading or learning in schools must undergo a thorough eye examination. Refraction is a signifant area of ocular examination, and must be done with cycloplegia. Eye examination should also include a careful assessment of ocular motility, especially phorias and convergence.

Needless to say, a fundus examination should be included in the eye checkup. Other than a meticulous eye examination, an MRI scan of brain should also be performed. Recently, researchers have found a link between the size of an area of brain involved in language processing. Since dyslexia also runs in families, though in varying severities, a genetic pre-disposition is also surmised.

Treatment Options

Dyslexia is not a disease. It is a developmental defect of brain. Similarly, there is no 'cure' of dyslexia, but there are, however, a range of specialist and well-targeted interventions that can help children improve their reading and writing skills. The sooner the child is diagnosed and receives specialist treatment, the better the chances of long-term improvement.

Psychological management of the child is also important. He or she should not feel that the problem will cause social embarrassment or they will be rebuked. Confidence building measures are also an integral part of treatment.

A teacher, who is specially trained in managing dyslexia, usually uses techniques involving taping into the faculties of touch, vision and hearing. Children are trained to improve the following skills:

1. Learning to understand phonemes
2. Reading out aloud
3. Vocabulary building
4. Reading comprehension.
5. Improving writing skills

A child is made to understand, by repeated practice, differences in letters and words, which where confusing previously. Gradually, by dedicated practise, children have overcome the disability to quite an extent.

Prognosis

In dyslexia, prognosis varies enormously. It affects such wide range of children, in a variety of ways, producing different symptoms of varying degrees that predicting individual outcome is extremely difficult.

Prognosis is better in children who are diagnosed early and receive appropriate expert treatment medically as well as psychologically.

Although, the outcome for children with dyslexia depends upon the severity of their disorder, but majority of them lead a normal, productive life.

DYSPRAXIA

Dyspraxia refers to difficulty with fine motor skills. Children with this defect will have problem in holding a pencil, picking neatly small objects, and problems in similar fine motor skills. The hand–eye coordination, which is so important in performing certain fine motor tasks, is underdeveloped.

DYSGRAPHIA

Dysgraphia refers to a disability or difficulty in writing or comprehending what is being said and synthesizing it into written material. Basic writing disorder consists of physical difficultly in forming letters and words. A more advanced disability indicates a struggle to organize thoughts on paper.

Symptoms of dysgraphia revolve around the act of writing. The salient features are:

1. Neatness and consistency of writing
2. Accurately copying letter and words
3. Spelling consistency
4. Organization in writing.

DYSCALKULIA

Learning disability in mathematics vary greatly depending on the child's other strengths and weaknesses. A child's ability in maths will also be affected by language learning disability, and visual defect or difficulty in sequencing memory or organizational cognitive abilities.

Basically, with a math-based learning disorder, a child may struggle memorization and organization of number or operational signs, e.g. a child may confuse between a 't' sign with a '×' multiplication sign and may express erroneouly with 5 + 5, and 5 × 5. Children with this defect may also have trouble counting certain numbers (like 2 or 5) or have difficulty in telling time.

DYSPHASIA

Language and communication disability involves the inability to understand or speak spoken language.

To produce a spoken language, one requires cognitive ability to think what to speak and organize it into proper words to express the thoughts. Some words may be pronounced incorrectly or missed while speaking.

Role of Vision Therapy

In 1998, the American Academy of Pediatrics, American Academy of Ophthalmology and American Association of Pediatric Ophthalmology and Strabismus (AAPOS) issued a policy statement regarding the use of 'vision therapy', specifically for the treatment of 'learning problems and dyslexia'.

Though there is a strong relationship between visual and perceptual problems, eye exercises used in behavioural vision therapy, also known as developmental optometry, are practiced by certain optometrists. Behavioural vision therapy aims to treat problems including difficulties of 'visual attention and concentration', which may manifest as an inability to sustain focus or to shift focus from one area to another area in space rather rapidly. Some of exercises described are:

1. Marsden balls

2. Rotation trainers
3. Syntonics
4. Balance beams
5. Saccadic fixates
6. Directional sequencers.

These exercises do not have any relation to improvement of vision but are taken as 'perceptual motor activities', being in the sphere of speech therapy or occupational therapy. They are aimed to basically improve motor skills and help a person certain motor tasks. There has been a strong opposition to the practice of so-called 'vision therapy' in treatment of behavioural problems. The AAO and AAPOS almost declared war on behavioural optometry condemning the therapy and its contention. Even within the field of optometry—where this is practiced, noted 'continuous absence of rigorous scientific evidence to support vision therapy practices'. Furthermore, vision problems are not the basis for learning disabilities.

Ineffective, controversial methods of treatment, such as 'vision therapy', may give parents and teachers a false sense of security that a child's disorder is being addressed, may waste time and delay proper instruction or mediation.

CONCLUSION

Learning disorders are a wide variety of disabilities a child may represent. Most of them mimic, at least in early stages, as visual problems. Dyslexia, in particular, shows strong resemblance to vision deficit. A child copies wrong letters from the blackboard or spells out incorrectly while reading, and thus strong suspicion arises of vision defect. Therefore, it is understandable that parents will bring the child to an ophthalmologist for evaluation. At this juncture, the eye specialist should be very careful to differentiate between an actual vision defect or something else. Where, in fact, refractive error is detected, a proper spectacle correction should be prescribed. Even then, if the problem is not resolved, then a strong suspicion of learning disability should arise and appropriate referral done.

A child psychologist or a speech therapist is the proper person for further management.

It should be also noted that in cases of amblyopia, the child may spell wrongly 'c' as 'o'; or 'k' as 'x'. But there would not be 'reversal' of letters, as explained above. As vision improves with treatment in amblyopia, the reading would attain normalcy.

Colour Vision

Colour vision is one of the most important of visual functions and is comparable to the loss of visual acuity. Children, who are born colour blind, have the same difficulty in learning and overall development as would occur if they were visually handicapped. In the early development in school age, children learn about the world with the colours which abound around them; in classes, they learn to paint, draw, and play with coloured objects. When they find they cannot do what other normal children are doing—even to the extent of being rebuked—they suffer psychologically and their mental development also suffers. Therefore, this part of visual function is being taken as seriously as other important visual functions, and will be dealt in detail here.

GENERAL CONDITIONS

Colour 'blindness' is an inaccurate term. It is a perceptual insensitivity to certain colours or inability to see colours accurately, and thus a more precise term would be 'colour vision deficiency' (CVD). Though, in most extreme form, no colour could be recognizable and this condition is extremely rare and is associated with severe congenital disease.

Red-green defect is the most common form and comprises of almost 99% of all cases, and causes problems in differentiating red and green colours.

Red colour defect is known as protanopia and has varied severity. Children may still recognize some shades of red but

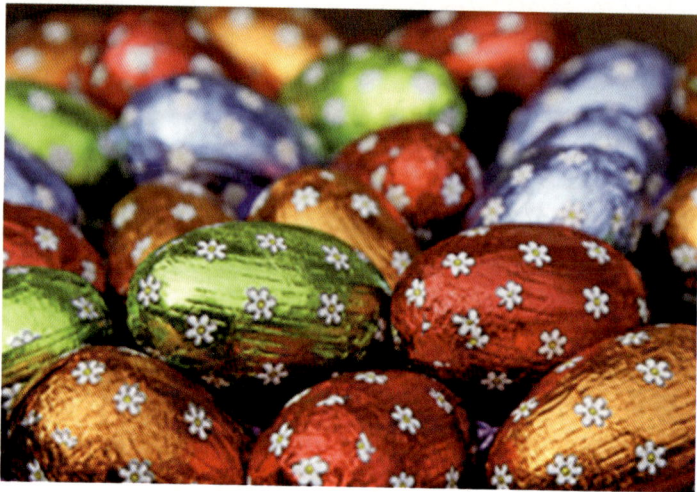

Fig. 11.1: Detection of colour objects in a normal person

not subtle hues; 'bright' red may not be recognized but some shades towards darker can be seen. Such disparity is labelled as 'protanomalous' colour defect.

Green colour defect is called 'deuteranopia' and in partial severity, called 'deuteraomalous' defects.

Similarly, unable to identify blue colour is labelled as 'tritanopia', and in partial form termed as 'tritanomalous' defects.

Total lack of any colour perception or 'colour blindness' is extremely rare and termed as 'Achromatopsia'. Colour vision is only in shades of grey.

Another form of rare colour defect is called 'unilateral dichromacy', affecting people who have one normal eye and other colour blind eye.

The red-green defect is more predominant due to the fact that red and green pigment genes involved in colour vision are located on the X-chromosome (Fig. 11.2).

Racial and ethnic differences have also been noted. The prevalence is more in white Caucasian races (5–6%); Asian (3–4%); Hispanics (2–3%); and in black races (1–2%).

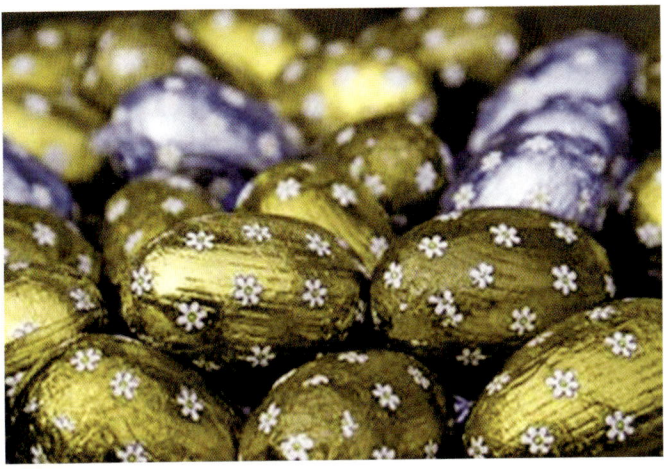

Fig. 11.2: Appearance of coloured objects with red-green defect

Males (boys) are more affected about 3–4% of total population and 0.3% in females.

Colour deficiency is a hereditary condition. The trait is passed on the X chromosome and because males have only one X chromosome, it is easier for them to inherit the disease.

A mother who carries one normal X chromosome and one X chromosome with the defective or mutant gene with red or green pigment, is not affected. But her son has a 50% chance of having the colour defect. Fathers cannot pass the defective gene as they transmit only the Y chromosome; but they can pass the defective X chromosome to their daughters, who while carrying the gene, do not manifest the disease. For a woman to inherit the colour vision defect, she must have a mother who is a 'carrier' and a father who has the colour 'defect'. This combination is rare and hence the far less defect in girls.

As discussed in previous chapters, the colour vision matures with the maturation of fovea, that is, around 6 months of age. By this age, an infant is able to recognize primary colours. But the full function of fovea with visual acuity reaching to normal VA of 6/6 is around 4 years. Therefore, it is generally agreed that proper colour vision testing should be done after 4 years of age.

Colour defect can also be 'acquired', not only by diseases of macula and optic nerve but also due to exposure to toxins or certain drugs. Macular dystrophies, retinitis pigmentosa, optic neuritis, leber hereditary optic atrophy, leber amaurosis, and related retinal diseases affecting macula. Stroke, head injury to occipital cortex, and multiple sclerosis (MS) affect colour vision.

Heavy metal poisoning, anti-malarials, antipsychotic drugs, and hydroxychloroquine, affect colour vision. These injure the visual acuity also; and the colour defect improves with the recovery from the disease.

Acquired colour defects may also arise in the following conditions: Glaucoma, diabetes, Alzheimer's disease, parkinsonism, chronic alcoholism, leukaemia, and sickle cell anaemia.

HOW DO WE SEE COLOURS!

We perceive the natural light as 'white' although it is actually a mixture of colours spanning from deep blue to deep red. This spectrum of colours depends upon the wavelength of each colour. Since they are mixed together, the spectrum appears white; and if we break the spectrum into different wavelength by suitable means, the seven-colour spectrum is demonstrated.

Let's see an example of a 'strawberry'. Most of us see it as red but do we all see the 'same' red? We will discuss this difference in 'hues' of a colour later in this chapter. Strawberries and other coloured objects reflect some wavelengths of light and absorb others. It is the reflected light that we perceive as colours! A strawberry appears red because its surface is reflecting only longer wavelength red light and absorbing other wavelengths. An object appears 'white' because it is reflecting 'all' the colour wavelengths, which mixed together appears white, as in natural light.

And a 'black' object appears black as it absorbs all the light and reflects none.

In a fully developed retina, there are 120 million rods and 6 million cones. Both contain photosensitive pigment that undergoes chemical change when they absorb light. This chemical change acts like a 'on-switch', triggering electrical signals which are passed from the retina to the visual cortex.

It should be remembered that rods contain only one photo-pigment while cones contain three types of photopigment, viz; red, green and blue, specific for each cone.

It is interesting to note that humans are the only mammals to possess three different types of photopigment. Other species of mammals have only two types of pigment. Butterflies have more than three pigments; they can perceive colours which we can only imagine! Since the eyes and brain together translate light into colours, there can occur slight differences in perception of colours. Your blue may not be the same blue as mine or in case of colour defect your red and green may appear brown to me.

HISTORY

One of the earliest methods used to test colour vision was to compare the indivisual's colour naming with that of a normal person. This was the standard method employed by Tuberville since 1684!

Dalton in 1798 gave a detailed description of his own colour perceptions, being himself a protanope! The next advancement in testing was made by Seeback in 1837, who required the subjects to choose from a wide-range of colour samples and match them with selected test samples. Variants of this method was subsequently used by other researchers, using different colour samples. More than 150 years have elapsed since then but his ingenious method, though modified, is still in use today.

Helmholtz in 1866 was the first person to hypothesise that colour blindness could manifest in three forms—red, green, or violet, depending upon the missing type of colour receptor in eyes.

Based on this hypothesis, Holmgren's wool test was introduced in 1877.

The idea of colour recognition by colour mixing was first introduced by Stilling in 1873. The success of this test depends upon the ability of colour defective individuals to discriminate between certain colours. A symbol (letter, number, or figure) composed of certain colour spots is set in a background of differently coloured spots. The design of template involves colours chosen so that the symbol is not recognized by a colour defective person. This forms the basis of the hugely popular 'pseudo-isochromatic' tests design. The name pseudo-isochromatic is derived from the concept that the symbol is 'falsly' appearing of the same colour as the background, hence not visible.

Lord Rayleigh in 1881, using his colour mixing apparatus, discovered that colour 'mixing' was different in several observers which were part of assumed 'normal' subjects. It is generally agreed that perception of 'hues' in colours varies in even normal subjects. A 'bright red' may not appear as bright to another person; a bright green to one person may appear to be dull green to another person. The spectral colours (natural colours in spectrum) used for mixing by Rayleigh, was incorporated in Nagel's Anomaloscope in 1907. It is universally agreed that Anomaloscope is the only clinical method capable of classifying colour defects in most accurate way.

SIGNS AND SYMPTOMS

To identify whether a child is colour defective, a simple colour game at home can help. On a sheet of white paper, colour an area of about 2 cm by 2 cm of colours red, green, orange, brown, blue, purple and grey. The coloured areas can be randomly placed but red, green and brown should be placed adjacent to each other. Show the paper in normal light and ask the child to name the coloured areas. If the child says that he/she is not sure whether the colours are red, green, or brown, then the child is red-green defective should be suspected. If the child says that the colours appear as pink or orange, then also red-green defect should be suspected.

Milder forms of colour deficiency are more common and many children never realize that they have any colour problem.

The following points should be looked into while assessing a child being colour defective:

- A child may look at colours differently than normal children. A bright red may be of dull red hue or some other shade.
- Stating or using wrong colours while copying. For example, using purple colour for green leaves on a tree.
- Difficulty in choosing colours for drawing.
- Low attention when colouring on a work sheet.
- Denial of colour issues.
- Copying wrong colours.
- Problem in identifying red or green colour pencils or any colour pencil having red or green component like brown or purple.
- Smelling of food before eating as colour of vegetables or food products cannot be identified.
- Difficulty in identifying colours in dim light.
- Excellent sense of smell.
- Excellent night vision.
- Children may complain that their eyes or head hurts when looking at bright red or green.
- When selecting red or green blocks, a child may complain that there are 'no' red or green blocks given to him, only purple or blue.
- Usually, except severe colour defects, visual acuity is not affectcd.

TYPES OF COLOUR DEFECTS

As already mentioned, the three types of cone carry three different colour photopigments, i.e. red, green and blue. These are also called the 'primary colour pigments'. The identification of colours in nature depends upon how much the different colour cones are stimulated (Fig. 11.3).

The type of colour blindness depends upon which type of cone is defective. The defect also varies in intensity. Subtle defects in the photopigments give rise to milder forms of colour defects and thus are not labelled as 'colour blind'.

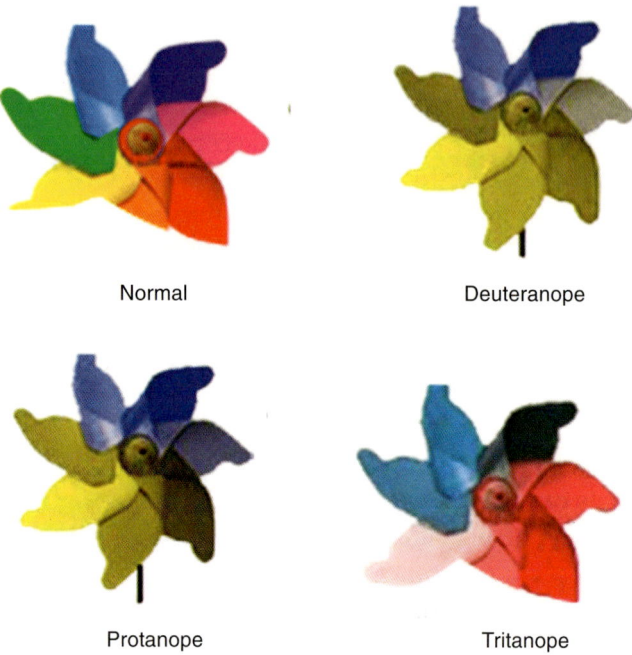

| Normal | Deuteranope |
| Protanope | Tritanope |

Fig. 11.3: Appearance of colours in 3 types of colour defects

Based on the above principles, the following classification, if followed.

1. *Protanomaly:* In protanomaly, the red cone photopigment is abnormal. Red, orange, and yellow appear greener and colours perceived are not as bright. In milder forms, 'protanomalous' children work normally and the condition does not interfere with daily life (Fig. 11.4B).

   In severe form, known as 'protanopia', where red colour pigment is totally deficient, red appears as black! Other shades of red, green and orange appear yellow. The incidence of male protanopia is about 1%.

2. *Deuteranomaly:* This is a green cone pigment defect. In milder forms, known as 'deuteranomaly', yellow and green appear redder and it is difficult to distinguish between violet and blue. Deuteranomalous children, which have the milder form

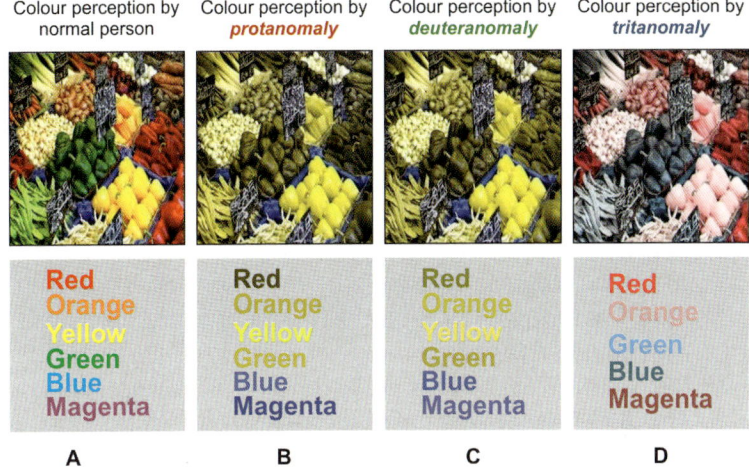

Colour perception by normal person	Colour perception by *protanomaly*	Colour perception by *deuteranomaly*	Colour perception by *tritanomaly*
Red Orange Yellow Green Blue Magenta	Red Orange Yellow Green Blue Magenta	Red Orange Yellow Green Blue Magenta	Red Orange Green Blue Magenta
A	**B**	**C**	**D**

Fig. 11.4: Colour preception by (A) Normal person, (B) protanomaly, (C) deuteranomaly, (D) tritanomaly

of disease, can function quite normally, without even noticing the defect. Deuteranomaly is the commonest form of X-linked colour defect, affecting 5% of males (Fig. 11.4C).

In severe form called 'deuteranopia', there are no working green cones. Affected children see yellow and green as 'beige'. Deuteranopia is also X-linked, affecting about 1% of males.

3. *Tritanomaly:* This is a blue cone photopigment disorder, often termed as blue–yellow defect. This is the least prevalent of all three defects and is extremely rare. Blue appears green and yellow towards pink shade (Fig. 11.4D).

In severe forms called 'tritanopia', there is no pigment in blue cones and blue appears green and yellow as violet.

This is an autosomal recessive disorder and appears in males and females equally.

4. *Complete colour blindness:* Children with total colour blindness called 'monochromacy' don't experience colour at all and visual acuity is also affected.

There are two types of colour monochromacy—cone monochromacy and rod monochromacy.

a. *Cone monochromacy:* This is a rare form of colour defect and is present since birth. Only one form of colour cone is functioning, so there would be red cone monochromacy; green cone monochromacy; and blue cone monochromacy. Since brain requires at least two basic colours to mix and compare signals from different colour cones to recognise colour, there is trouble in recognising various colours. Cone monochromacy is an autosomal recessive disorder.

b. *Rod monochromacy:* This is also known as 'acromatopsia'. This is also a rare autosomal recessive disorder. Here none of the three cone pigments are present and is the most severe form of colour blindness.

It is a congenital defect and children see their world as black or in shades of grey. Bright light causes photophobia and children prefer to work in dim light. Children have poor visual acuity, amblyopia, and nystagmus.

ETIOPATHOGENESIS

The three types of photopigment cone cells work together; but each is stimulated differently according to the wavelengths of colours present in the incident light, and the brain then realizes the colours as what we see. For example, when blue and red cones are stimulated in a certain way, we see purple colour.

Inherited colour defects are caused by abnormal or defective photopigments. These colour detecting molecules are present in the cone cells of the photoreceptive layer of retina. It has been found that several genes are needed to produce photopigments and defects or mutations in these genes lead to the colour defects.

Genes are bundled together in chromosomes. One copy of each chromosome is passed by the parent at conception through egg and sperm. The X and Y chromosomes known as sex chromosomes determine whether the baby born will be male (XY) or female (XX).

In X-linked inheritance, the mother carries the defective or mutated gene on one of her X chromosome and will pass on that gene to 50% of her children. Since females have two X chromosomes, the effect of one defective gene is counteracted by the normal gene on the other chromosome. Thus in such cases, the female child will not be affected but will remain as carrier.

Now if mother is affected (carrier) and father unaffected, the following situations can present:

a. There is 50% chance that a son will have the disorder.

b. 50% chance that a daughter will be carrier.

c. No chance that any daughter will have the disease.

In autosomal recessive inheritance, it takes two copies of the mutant gene to give rise to the disease. An individual who has one copy of the mutant gene, is said to be a 'carrier'. When two carriers have a child, the following situations arise:

a. 50% chance of child being a carrier.

b. 25% chance of a child having the disease.

c. 25% chance of a child neither being a carrier nor a sufferer.

In autosomal dominant inheritance, it takes just one copy of the mutant gene to transmit the disease. If one parent has 'mutant dominant' gene, there is 50% chance of a child having the disease.

IMPLICATIONS OF COLOUR BLINDNESS

Normal identification of various colours is a vital part of our daily life. Severe colour defect is a serious disability and hinders the normal development of a child. The list of implications of a severely handicapped child is unending and self explanatory.

The important issues are related to vocations and employments which require sharp colour vision like pilots, railway and road drivers, security services.

Professionals like artists, architects, and even doctors are affected. Medical surgeons will not be able to detect the colour of blood, when oxygen saturation drops. Grocery vendor will not know the colour of a ripe banana, or a red tomato will appear green to him.

Beauticians in parlours will not understand the red colour of lipstick and will apply purple colour instead!

These are some examples which affect numerous professions in daily life.

DESCRIPTION OF COLOUR VISION TESTS

Over the years, several different kinds of tests have been generated to detect colour defects. They are based on certain principles but the basic aim is to detect the type of colour defect and to quantify to the best extent possible.

The tests envisage detecting a particular colour amidst a background multiple colours (pseudo-isochromatic tests); matching of a colour given with standard samples of colours (the anomaloscopes, 100-hue tests, etc.); or simply detect the different hues of colours presented to the subject (lantern tests).

All have their importance depending upon the age of the person, the specificity required, the time consumed, understanding of the person about the test, only screening purpose or quantification and so on.

PSEUDO-ISOCHROMATIC TESTS

There are different types of pseudo-isochromatic tests but the most common and prevalent is the Ishihara plates. This will be dealt in detail, rest will be given a passing note. Some tests are not commercially available, and hence are omitted. All provide efficient screening (90–95% specificity) of red–green and blue–yellow colour defect. Basically these tests consist of a series of plates or cards on which coloured dots of various sizes are printed to form a figure of shades of specific colour against a background of multicoloured dots. The figure is in the form of a letter, numerical or a geometrical configuration like circle, triangle or cross.

An important aspect of these plates and a word of caution is that these plates are designed to be viewed only under standard conditions of illumination, i.e. normal sun light. Viewing under tungsten bulb will give yellow light and fluorescent tube will give white light. Both do not conform to sunlight.

There are certain disadvantages as well. Firstly, the illumination has to be kept in mind as this will give inconsistent results when the test is done in room light. Secondly, the success of test depends upon choosing appropriate 'confusing colours', which are still not optimum. Third, tests should be used primarily as screening test to divide persons into normal and colour defective population only. In any case, these are good tool to identify children who are red or green defective.

The Ishihara Plates

As is the trend in this book to honour the luminaries who have contributed to the development of medical science, a brief resume will be given of inventor of this test as a tribute to him.

Dr Shinobu Ishihara (1879–1963), while working in the military medical school, was asked to devise a test to screen military recruits for abnormalities of colour vision. His assistant was a colour defective physician who helped him to test the various plates devised by Dr Ishihara.

The original test consisted of collection of 38 plates filled with coloured dots which forms the base of the test. The dots are coloured in different colour shades and a numerical number is hidden inside of another colour.

The original test has gone under several modifications with an attempt to choose the right background colours to create enough confusion to identify the hidden figure. Also 'hidden wavy lines' have been added for use in the illiterate population and small children (Fig. 11.5).

In all modified editions, plate 1 is the demonstration plate. It consists of a double-digit numerical formed by small coloured circles appearing on a background of different colour circles. If an observer misses the demonstration plate, the test should be discontinued. The remaining plates are based on pseudo-isochromatic principle, i.e. the dots or circles to the colour defective person will 'look alike', but are not actually so.

The number of plates varies with the edition. For 38-plate book, plates 1 to 21 are for screening red–green defect; and

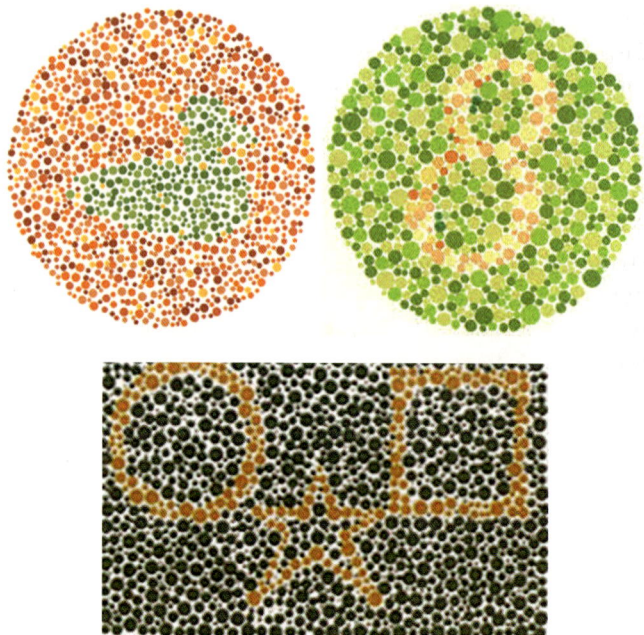

Fig. 11.5: Ishihara colour plates for children.

plates 22 to 25 are for differential diagnosis of protan from deutan. The remainder plates are for illiterates.

For mass screening, the test may be shortened by using plate 1, one plate each from 2 to 5, 6 to 9, 10 to 14, 15 to 17 and 18 to 21.

In 24 plate edition, plate 1 is demonstration plate, plates 2 to 14 for screening and 16–17 for differentiation of protan and deutan; and rest for illiterates.

In 16-plate edition, plates 2 to 9 for screening, plate 10 for differentiation and rest for illiterates.

More recently, plates for children have been introduced, which have geometrical designs or toy-shaped figures.

Procedure: The subject is instructed to read the numerical within '3 seconds'. The plates are held at reading distance and to be read in 'day light'. The plates are numbered. No record sheet is provided but scoring instructions accompany the test.

In 38-plate edition, less than 4 errors are within normal limit. In 24-plate and 16-plate editions, 2 or less errors are permissible. As of reliability or specificity, Ishihara plates are considered as one of the best screening tests.

Remark: The test is very useful for rapid screening of red–green colour defects. It provides good, reliable diagnosis of protans and deutans and classifies moderate to severe level of defects. No tritan plates are available. The Ishihara plate test is the most widely used test all over the world and with the incorporation of toy figures, it has become a very valuable test for children as well.

Other Tests Based on Pseudo-Isochromatic Plates

1. *Standard Pseudo-Isochromatic plates:* This test was designed by Ishikawa, Hukani and Tanabe. In these plates, numericals are formed by a specific colour dots on a background of multicoloured dots based on vanishing design. Here all plates have numericals only.

2. *Tokyo Medical College test:* This test was designed to screen red–green and blue–yellow defect as well. The test consists of double-digit numericals. The test is based on the pseudo-isochromatic plates. The test has an instruction manual and a scoring sheet. There are 5 screening plates for red–green defect and 2 for blue–yellow defect. These are then followed by 3 plates to differentiate red (protan) from green (deutan) defective persons. And 3 more to estimate the severity of red-green defect.

   Remark: The test is a good for rapid screening of both red–green as well as blue–yellow defects with fair accuracy. Though the severity can be detected but 'anomalous' defects cannot be ascertained. Also the plates are not optimally pruned to detect tritans (blue defect).

3. *Hardy-Rand-Rittler test:* The H-R-R test, as is commonly known, was introduced by LeGrand Hardy, Gertude Rand and Catherine Rittler. The test is based on pseudo-isocromatic plates. Since the test is not commercially available, it will not be discussed here.

4. *Dvorine test:* The test was devised by Dr Israel Dvorine and is based on pseudo-isochromatic plates and is used to screen red and green defects. The test consists of single and double numericals (15 plates) and coloured 'paths' to be traced. Scoring sheet is provided.

   The first plate is the demonstration plate. Rest are all test plates and consist of coloured circle on a background of multicoloured circles. The colours size is so chosen that it can be well read with VA better than 6/60.

   Twelve are screening plates and plates no. 6 and 7 are diagnostic plates.

   Classification of severity is based on the number of plates missed. That is missing 0–2 is normal; 3–4 indicates mild defect; 5–11 indicates moderate defect and missing 12–14 indicates severe defect. The advantage over other tests is that scoring sheet is provided and quantitatively the severity of the defect can be diagnosed.

5. *Titmus pediatric colour perception test:* This is based on the pseudo-isochromatic plates of colour confusion. The test consists of a slide projected at 20 ft., by a Titmus vision screener and is viewed binocularly through a stereoscope.

   The slide contains eight blocks of coloured dots, in which an 'E' of a colour is embedded. The child is expected to indicate the direction in which the arms of E are pointing, if the coloured E is recognised.

   Errors of 3 or more are considered as failure.

   Remark: No validation or reliability data are available. It may be considered a gross colour vision screener and the test has to be validated by an Ishihara 'line' or 'figure' plate for children.

6. *Chalk colour test for children:* This test was developed by Dr Guilherme Martins from Brazil and is usually applied in children ranging from age 6 to 12. The test consists of matching chalk pieces of different colours with a chalk piece of a fixed colour. The test is user friendly as children are more accustomed to chalk pieces. The test has 100% specificity and 50% sensitivity. According to this test, male

children incidence was found to be 2.6% and female child incidence 0.9%.

Arrangement or Matching Tests

In these tests, the person is required to arrange coloured samples by similarity or match them in a sequential colour series.

This kind of test was developed by Pierce in 1934 and was first used in National Institute of Industrial Psychology in London.

Pseudo-isochromatic tests are used to separate colour defective subjects from normal persons, but cannot specify subtle differentiation of 'hues' of the same colour, as wide range of colour differentiation ability and aptitude exists in normal subjects. These tests not only identify colour defective individuals but also identify the 'anomalous' colour defects.

In Pierce's original test, there were two types of procedures. In the grading procedure, 16 discs of one colour were presented to the observer who had to arrange them in a specified saturation series. In the matching procedure, pre-arranged discs of one colour but of different 'hues' or shades were presented to the person, who then had to select their match from a duplicate set of discs given to him.

Modern variants were devised by Farnsworth in 1943 in the Farnsworth–Munsell 100 hue test and the Farnsworth D-15 test.

1. *Farnsworth-Munsell 100 hue test:* The test became commercially available in 1949 and is continuing till date and widely used all around the world.

   The colours are mounted in small caps or disc-shaped holders and arranged in fixed order, and labelled at the back. 25 holders are arranged in one row of red, blue, green and yellow. The caps or holders are arranged in a specific order of changing hue of one colour which are put in a rectangular long box and packed in a carrying box which is portable (Fig. 11.6). There are 25 holders in each of 4 rows, hence the name '100-hue test'. The holders are removed from the box and the subject is asked to 'arrange' them in a fixed order of

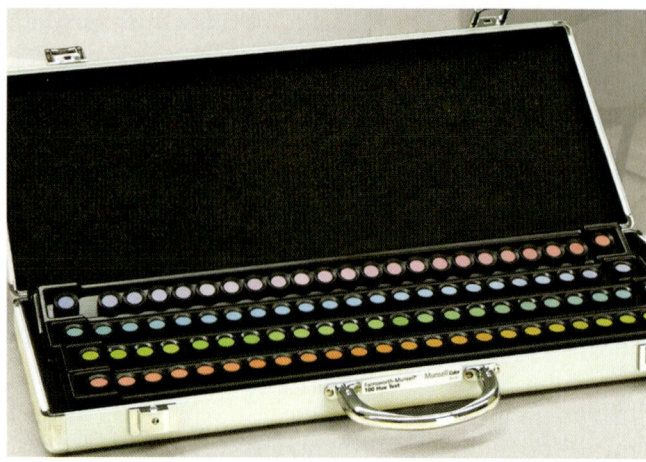

Fig. 11.6: Box of Farnsworth-Munsell colour test

hues, mentioned in the instruction manual and explained to the subject.

The test is time consuming and not very helpful for children. But is a simple and excellent test to detect anomalous individuals (Figs 11.6 and 11.7).

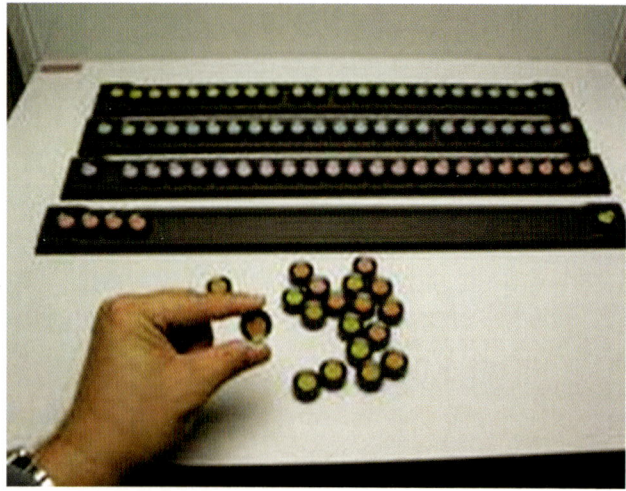

Fig. 11.7: Fransworth–Munsell colour test

A shortened version of this test is also available as Panel-D15 test which has 15 caps in each row.

In the present form, the test consists of 85 caps or holders in each of 4 rows in the carrying box.

2. *Anomaloscope:* Anomaloscopes are optical instruments in which the observer manipulates stimulus control knobs to match two coloured fields in given colour and brightness. The anomaloscope is the most standardized instrument for diagnosis of colour defects and its anomalous forms.

The principle is based on Rayleigh equation which specifies the combination of spectral colours (7 colours in the natural spectrum) to match a given colour.

Nagel's anomaloscope (Fig. 11.8): This is the most widely used anomaloscope. It consists of a viewing optical tube and the observer sees a lower half circle in the viewing field of a 'fixed colour'. The other top half contains combination of

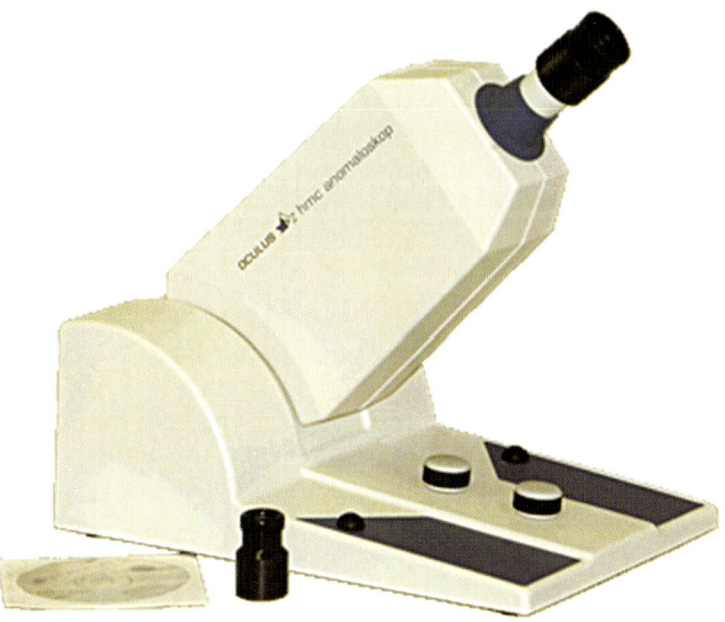

Fig. 11.8: Nagel's anomaloscope.

colours, which can be adjusted with a knob to match the colour given in the lower half. For example, the lower half has yellow colour of certain hue and brightness, and the observer manipulates the knob which mixes red and green colour in proportions to match the yellow colour hue in lower half. (Mixture of red and green gives yellow colour.)

The instrument is difficult to use and needs a technician specially trained to operate the equipment. Owing to the cumbersome technicality, the instrument is mostly used for research purpose.

3. *City university test:* This test is based on the colour matching principle and is designed to screen moderate to severe colour defective persons. Protans, deutans and tritans can be detected with this test. The test consists of 11 plates, each plate having 5 coloured circles—one central, surrounded by 4 comparison circles. The first plate is only demonstration plate. The remaining are test plates.

The observer must indicate which of the 4 coloured circles (top, bottom, right or left) most closely resembles the central test circle. The response has to be within 3 seconds. The plates are viewed at 35 cm and in 'daylight illumination'. Of the 10 plates, the response is circled under one of the four columns: Normal, protan, deutan, and tritan.

The test is a good, quick test and children over 5 years can undertake the test in reasonable way.

Lantern Tests

Lantern tests have been designed as the most practical way of identifying colours in different shades or hues.

The concept of lantern tests is quite simple, as they do not incorporate complex optical systems nor the use of complicated colour confusing or matching printed plates. Lantern tests simply require the identification of 'coloured lights' as is the requirement in daily life in day as well as night-time.

Therefore, this has become the most practical mode of testing colour defects for train drivers, bus drivers or pilots—who require identification of colours in day and night-time.

Different types of lantern tests have evolved like Giles-Archer, Edridge-Green, Martins, Sloan and Farnsworth lantern tests.

Edridge-Green lantern test: **This** most commonly used lantern test designed to produce range of colours and tints. Seven coloured and seven modifying glass filters and seven apertures are used in the apparatus. The coloured filters represent the seven spectral colours and the modifying filters represent smoke, fog, rain, mist, clouds, dim light, and bright light. The aperture sizes can be varied and represent the coloured lights to be viewed from varying distances (Fig. 11.9).

The test is performed in a dark room from 20 feet distance. The colours are presented in a random order and the observer names the colour of light. The aperture can be changed in accordance with the requirement of working distance of the person.

Edridge-Green is a wonderful test devised for practical use in testing colour identification in different atmospheric conditions in many vocations where seeing red, green and yellow coloured lights are important.

The test was designed for a specific purpose and may or may not be very useful for children.

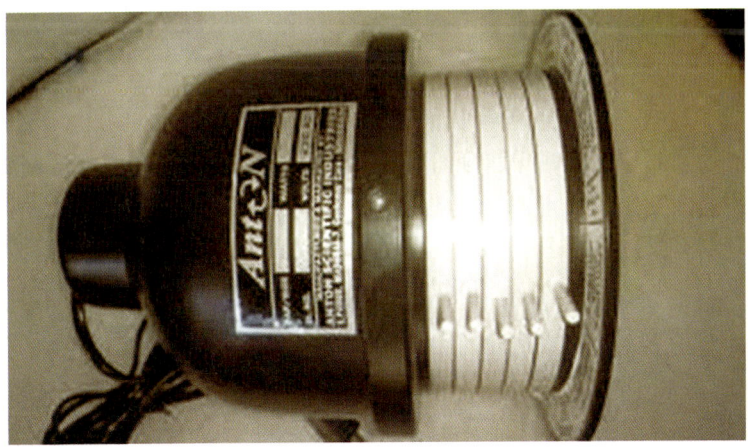

Fig. 11.9: Edridge-green lantern

CONCLUSION

As already stated, colour vision is very important in the normal mental and psychological development of children. Also if a child is found to be severely colour defective, then appropriate measures can be taken from the beginning to groom the child in a particular manner. Though no treatment is available for congenital colour blind children, but they are taught to recognize colours in a different way. And these children are primed to choose vocations where colour identification is not of significance.

Of all the various types of colour tests described here, none of them conforms for testing in a small child. Broadly speaking, children are not mature enough to identify colours before the age of 4 years. After that age, children can be tested for colour defects by the most simple way possible. Smart children do well with the Ishihara test plates, especially having line diagrams or toy figures.

Matching tests, particularly those with coloured circles or even simpler 'chalk matching' test can be used. The idea is to use a test which is child friendly and best suited for the intelligence level and cooperation of the child.

Contrast Sensitivity

In simple terms, contrast sensitivity means differentiating a given object from its background. We all can resolve and recognise objects of high contrast and in good illumination. But things around us are not always in high contrast. Visual perceptions change as background illumination changes, from broad daylight to twilight or more dim illumination. It is then that our visual system's efficiency is at stake. It is not differentiating only black and white, but change in illumination also affects the colour of objects from its background.

Apart from numerous diseases of eyes and brain which affect the contrast sensitivity, there are inherent individual variations in contrast sensitivity.

It is now generally agreed that visual acuity measures only one aspect of visual function, which analyses the clarity of vision, the finest detail which a human eye can resolve. But contrast sensitivity not only measures the acuity but the clarity of vision at all levels of illumination. Thus this is supposed to be more complete analysis of visual function in our day-to-day life.

The conventional method of testing or the most widely used index of sight, the visual acuity, is a measure of our spatial resolving power. Our world, which we inhabit, is packed with different patterns and colours of varying intensity. Therefore, objects viewed in everyday life vary, in intensity or luminance, quite unlike the fixed, high contrast optotypes traditionally found in charts of Snellen type.

The clinical relevance of visual sensitivity to contrast was first appreciated a century back! But its importance was not understood and its use did not become widespread.

A practical test of visual contrast sensitivity was first developed in 1918; but was not put to commercial use. A true understanding of this feature of vision was shown by innovative studies of Campbell and colleagues in 1960 at Cambridge. Two aspects of their work gained credence. Firstly, the intuitive finding that how we are able to see in low illumination that in varying illumination, targets of 'medium' resolution are seen better than those of low or high resolution (Fig. 12.1), which came to be termed as 'contrast sensitivity function' (CSF). This discovery led to the notion that testing contrast sensitivity over a range of target resolutions (spatial frequencies) provides a more comprehensive and more sensitive evaluation of spatial visual function than simple visual acuity.

Secondly, the contrast sensitivity function appeared to be subserved by a series of neural channels, each responding to detail of a relatively narrow size range. Damage within the visual pathway might selectively inhibit sensitivity within one or more channels. Armed with this new 'tool' to assess visual function in a comprehensive way and which, in theory, had the potential to reveal anomalies of visual function so far undocumented, researchers developed a plethora of practical tests for contrast sensitivity. The most relevant queries which rose among clinicians was—'in what ocular conditions is contrast sensitivity affected and in what manner?' With a wave of tests, loss of contrast sensitivity was associated ranging from radial keratectomy to renal failure!

Several studies support the contention that contrast sensitivity function (CSF) gives a better evaluation of visual performance than Snellen test. It has been also found that patient's cerebral lesions who complaining of visual problems, often had severely abnormal CSF but normal Snellen acuity. In multiple sclerosis (MS), reduced CSF is the first sign than any other visual disturbance, hence its importance in diagnosing the disease early in younger persons.

DESCRIPTION OF CONTRAST SENSITIVITY TESTS

Reduced contrast sensitivity creates problems in driving, difficulty in recognizing people in dim light, tiring of eyes more easily while reading or watching TV. Poor contrast sensitivity also increases the risk of falling, if you fail to see steps in same coloured pavement or steps of different colour.

As far as children are concerned, many of the above problems can exist especially early tiring of eyes, dark adaptations, problem in negotiating steps, etc. The important issue of these visual problems is that so many children who have unilateral amblyopia are not aware of the loss of visual acuity but complain of certain asthenopic symptoms. In fact, in suspected cases of amblyopia, CSF is more reliable indicator of amblyopia.

In cases of retinitis pigmentosa, macular disorders, multiple sclerosis, recuperation from head injuries, etc. are some of the examples where contrast sensitivity testing is of paramount importance in diagnosing and following the disease process.

The most relevant application of CSF is in amblyopia in children. There are 2 sets of CSF response in amblyopia. Those with decreased sensitivity at all levels of spatial frequency and others with loss at higher frequencies only.

Pelli-Robson Test

The test was introduced by Dennis Pelli and John Robson in 1988. Like a standard Snellen chart, the Pelli-Robson chart consists of horizontal lines of Snellen optotypes in capital letters. But instead of the letters getting smaller in successive lines, it is the contrast of letters gradually diminishing against the white background. There are 8 lines of diminishing contrast. Each line consists of 6 letters of 6/18 size. Each line has two groups of 3 letters and these 3 letters in each group have the same contrast level. So there are 3 trials of same contrast level. The chart is wall mounted and viewed at one metre with standard illumination. The inference is done in log value of each line read.

The labelling starts from 00 in top line and has 0.4, 0.8, 1.2, 1.5, and 2.0 log values consecutively. A normal person should be able to identify contrast at line 1.5. Below this, the contrast is termed deficient.

Vistech (VCTS) 6000 and Vistech 6500 Test

Model 6000 is used for testing contrast at near while model 6500 is used for testing at distance of 10 feet. The test is based on the principle of sine-wave gratings of diminishing contrast, which makes it more valuable for testing in children also. Both test charts have 5 rows of increasing spatial frequencies, i.e. more cycles/degree, and in each row the contrast decreases from left to right. The lowest contrast grating identification is the CS value for that spatial frequency. The sensitivity at each spatial frequency can be used to plot a contrast sensitivity function (CSF) and can be compared with standard age norms provided with the test (*see* figure). There are at least half a dozen different varieties of contrast sensitivity charts, viz. Melbourne edge test, Berkeley glare test, Cambridge low contrast grating test, Mars hand-held CS test; but the most convenient and popular are the Pelli-Robson and Vistech tests which have been described in detail.

Out of these, Cambridge low contrast and Mars hand-held tests deserve some mention.

Cambridge low contrast test: The Cambridge test developed in 1989 has the advantage of being cheaper, easy to use and easy to interpret. The test measures CS at only one spatial frequency, i.e. 4 cycles/degree. It shows that when sensitivity to this spatial frequency is impaired, sensitivity at all frequencies is also impaired. It is performed at 6 metres distance and comprises of 12 plates with stripes of diminishing contrast. First plate is for demonstration, while rest test plates are numbered from 1 to 10. The plates are presented in normal room illumination sequentially from 1 to 10, till the patient fails to respond.

Mars hand-held test: The test was developed by Dr Aries Ardit in New York, USA, and unlike Pelli-Robson test, the letters are not arranged in triplets of equal contrast, instead each letter decreases in contrast by 0.04 log units. The contrast range is from 0.04 log units to 0.92 log units, in six lines. The advantage is that the chart is hand held and viewed at 40 cm and very easy for children as loss of attention at distance is obviated.

CONTRAST SENSITIVITY TESTING

In clinical practice, CS is generally measured by means of Optotypes of different contrast such as Pelli-Robson chart (Fig. 12.1) or by sinusoidal gratings of different spatial frequencies (Fig. 12.2). Since sinusoidal gratings are more standardized method of testing, the most popular commercial tests available are: (1) Functional acuity contrast sensitivity (FACT) test, and (2) Vector vision CSV-1000 test (Fig. 12.2). These tests commonly use 8 or 9 plates for each spatial frequency.

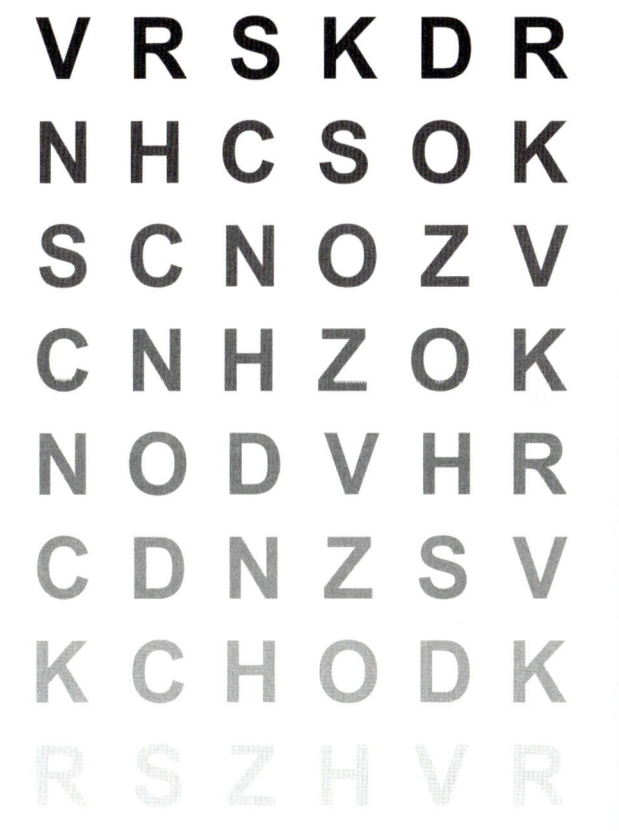

Fig. 12.1: Pelli-Robson chart—using the Snellen optotypes.

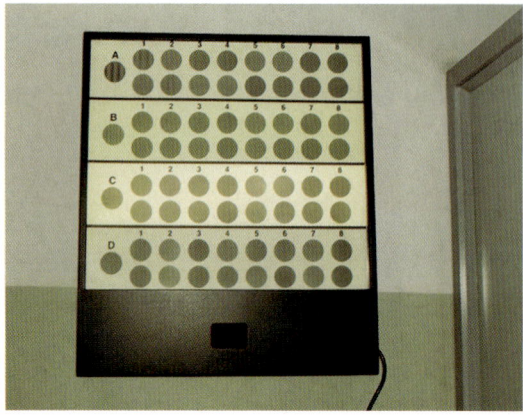

Fig. 12.2: Vector-vision test—USA (The above grating contrast sensitivity test is used at the author's clinic)

Recently, with advent of i-Pads, an i-Pad app has been developed by the brand name of 'Clinic CSF', where the CSF can be tested by portable means via the i-Pad.

Horizontal axis shows the 'spatial frequency ' of the bars, i.e. the number of bars or gratings presenting in one degree (Fig. 12.3).

Vertical axis shows diminution of 'contrast' between the black and white stripes, which measures from '1.0' (highest contrast) to '0' as the lowest contrast when the bars become invisible. The vertical meridian or contrast decreases by increments as 0.9, 0.8, 0.7, etc. up to 0.

The red parabolic line is the contrast sensitivity curve. It shows that the best contrast sensitivity is between 6 and 8 spatial frequency by the horizontal axis; and somewhere 0.2 contrast by the vertical axis, where the black bars become invisible.

It will be further observed that though the gratings are well spaced in smaller spatial frequencies, yet the sensitivity approaches its best mark where the frequency is between 6 and 8 cyl/deg., where the contrast is high. And then declines as the spatial frequency increases.

Similarly, with diminishing contrast between the bars, the sensitivity decreases and is the best at the peak of the curve.

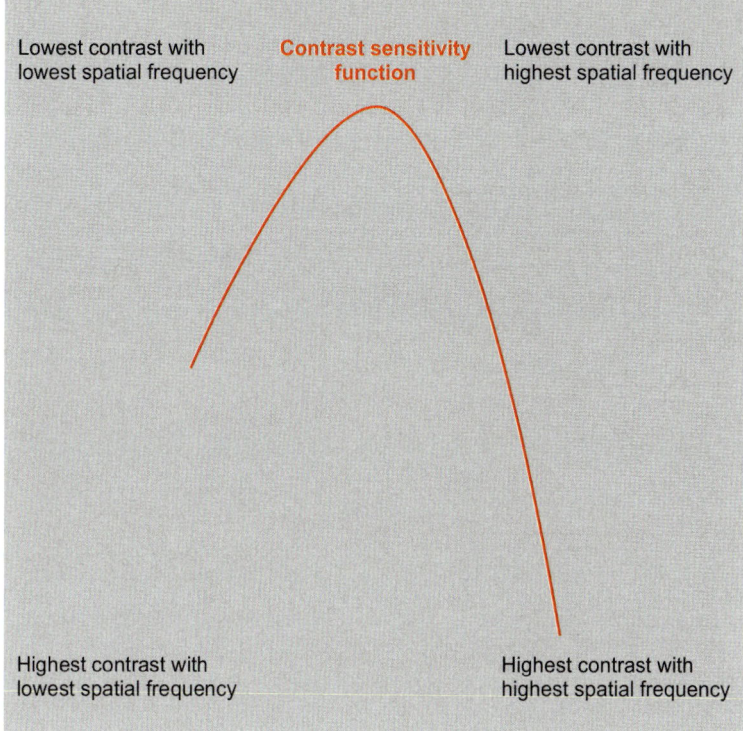

Lowest contrast with
lowest spatial frequency

**Contrast sensitivity
function**

Lowest contrast with
highest spatial frequency

Highest contrast with
lowest spatial frequency

Highest contrast with
highest spatial frequency

Fig. 12.3: Spatial frequency—cycles/degree (The above graph is the best depicted contrast sensitivity function).

It is also to be remembered that the contrast sensitivity increases gradually with age; from 2–3 cyl/degree in childhood to 6–8 cyl/degree by end of teenage.

It then gradually decreases with advancing age.

CONCLUSION

The above discussions amply purports the notion that contrast sensitivity is a better and more comprehensive method of evaluating the visual function of spatial sensitivity. In children, it is most relevant in assessing the improvement of amblyopia. It is also more sensitive tool in assessing recovery after head injuries, which are so common in children; in assessing improvements in number of childhood and adolescence cerebral disorders like multiple sclerosis, optic neuropathies, post-surgical tumours, etc. Over and above all these ailments, complaints of unexplained ocular asthenopia in children, where all routine tests show normal, contrast sensitivity must be tested.

Hyperacuity

The word 'acuity' or sharpness of vision has been pre-empted by centuries of association with the resolving power of eyes. In vision, it is embodied in the time-honoured '6/6' standard in eye charts, designed letters or figures of discernible 1 min/arc separation. But many spatial thresholds transcend this limit and a person is able to comprehend very fine discrepancies beyond this acuity limit. Vernier acuity is one such resolving power of the visual system to which the term 'hyperacuity' was first attached by Weistheimer in 1975.

Lately, some other examples of hyperacuity have been known which surpass the normal acuity. These are:

1. Curvature detection—judgement of deviations in contours.
2. Detection of sharpness or smoothness of edges.
3. Hyperstereocauity—fine detection of depth perception in three-dimensional objects.
4. Oscillatory movement displacement threshold.

Hyperacuity or 'super-resolution' is a term applied to a sensory capability that surpasses the limits of resolution power of retinal cone limits. Visual acuity, as well known, depends upon the distance between these light receptors, because their output is coded for only their own location and cannot be further subdivided. Established doctrine states visual acuity, as governed by retinal receptor spacing. The normal 1 min/arc roughly corresponds to the diameter of a single cone at the fovea and to distinguish two points or lines as separate,

3 cones have to be activated; the middle one spared or only lightly stimulated.

Though the sensory output is always funnelled through the retinal receptors, but information on structural differences in objects less than the spacing of elements of retinal mosaic can be extracted from activity pattern within an ensemble of other retinal elements. Hyperacuity, then, is the result of circuitry analysis of the inputs by the neurons in the brain that distils this information.

'Vernier alignment acuity' is a prime example of hyper-acuity. In the human fovea, two lines must be at least 1 min/arc apart to be seen as separate. But a misalignment of even 1/10th of this value can be detected by the visual cortex. This gives a hint of two kinds of neural processing. For acuity, two sensory peaks must be sufficiently sharp and far enough apart that the possibility of their overlap is minimized and differentiated excitation of at least 3 cones is assured. For Vernier acuity, it is the precision of location of each peak that matters (Fig. 13.1).

HYPERACUITY IN CHILDREN

Studies on the development of hyperacuity in children have been very informative. A study done comparing grating acuity and vernier acuity using visual-evoked potential showed that these two visual functions develop at similar rates from age one month to six years. After the age six, grating acuity becomes constant, but vernier acuity continues to improve, reaching

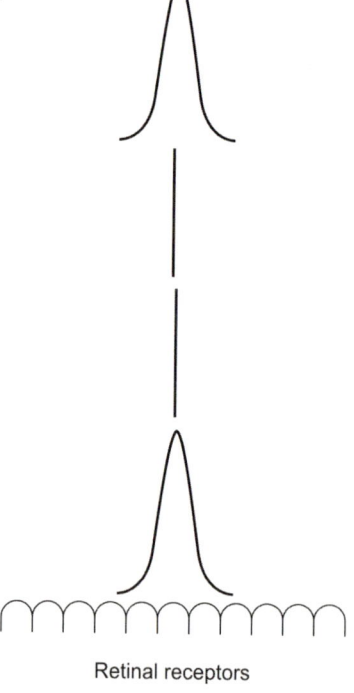

Retinal receptors

Fig. 13.1: Vernier acuity: The vertical lines are finely misaligned.

adult levels around 14 years of age. These results suggest that adult-like hyperacuity is not dependent upon grating or other types of visual acuity, and that development or plasticity of different visual performances are different at different ages.

Recognition of 'contour deformations' is another visual performance falling in the category hyperacuity. In number of significant studies, it has been found that in cases of amblyopia in children, contour difference identification is a more specific and predictive parameter to assess the progress in treatment. In strabismic amblyopia particularly, it has proved to identify amblyopia, assess progress of treatment and change of line of management.

The procedure consists of using circles of various diameter in degrees, i.e. 0.5 and 1.0 degree radius, with modulations on the ring having 8 modulations and 16 modulations on 360° circle. The diagrams can be used as charts (Fig. 13.2) for older children. For younger children, the paradigm of forced preferential looking test is used. Studies have been conducted in children ranging from 3 to 14 years. Studies on infants are not yet available. The results have proved this test to be more specific with 80% sensitivity for amblyopia management than Teller cards or Snellen charts.

Another visual function which comes in the domain of hyperacuity and has been used to detect and follow amblyopia recovery is 'ocsillatory movement displacement threshold' (OMDT). It is the smallest or faintest movement of a given stimulus which gives rise to the perception of movement. Even in cases where visual acuity has been found to be normal, visual deficits via OMDT have been used in glaucoma, diabetes, optic

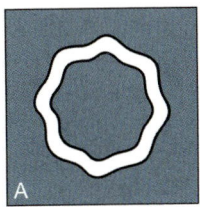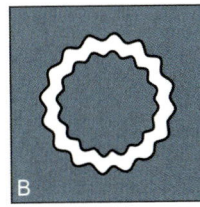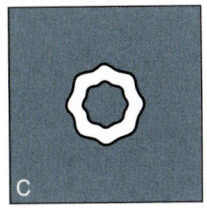

Fig. 13.2A to C: Contour deformity hyperacuity tests for amblyopia

neuropathies, amblyopia and other cerebral disorders in children.

In a study using the OMDT paradigm in amblyopic eyes, it was found that amblyopic eye had higher OMDT (25 sec/arc) than normal eye (18 sec/arc).

The importance of these hyperacuity visual functions is now well understood in cases of amblyopia in children and these are being used in some centres around the world. Amblyopia is usually measured in terms of visual acuity and its management progress also measured in terms of improvement of visual acuity. Though stereoacuity is now taken in normal protocol of amblyopia assessment but other hyperacuity functions are still not considered. Differences in the development patterns of variety of visual functions are well founded, but we have not used them to our advantage. Anatomically also, different parts of visual system display different degrees of maturation (plasticity). From retina to LGN to striate cortex, all show different periods of maturation. Even within the striate cortex, various layers subserving different functions mature at different ages. It may well be possible that a different sensitive period for normal development hyperacuity functions may exist and a permanent degradation of these functions may result while visual acuity, processed in a different area, may still be reversible. The whole idea of delving into different visual functions is to assess the plethora of functions our visual system possesses and know what goes wrong at different ages and ways and means to retrieve these functions again.

CONCLUSION

The disparity between visual acuity and other higher visual functions suggests that resolution acuity, used as a standard test of functional recovery, is unsuitable as an overall descriptor of amblyopia. Other measures, like contour abnormality and OMDT, may be more sensitive and predictive to neural damage and recovery than visual acuity alone, and may, therefore, describe visual loss not apparent from Snellen acuity.

Stereoacuity

Stereopsis is derived from a Greek word *stereo* meaning 'solid' and *opsis* meaning 'appearance'.

Stereo-vision or stereopsis or depth perception is based on the 'retinal image disparity', i.e. horizontal disparity of position of retinal images of objects between the two eyes. Stereoacuity, which is a measure of acuteness of this depth perception, provides an indication of the level of sensory binocularity an individual has. Stereopsis, therefore, is the highest degree of binocular vision, and represents one of the most important functions of the human vision. To a limited degree, stereoscopic vision is possible monocularly also involving monocular cues like size, shape, motion parallax, illumination difference, visual memory, etc. However, a completely missing or severe limitation of stereopsis is a severe handicap in many life-domains and vocations. This is the reason why this visual sense should be examined in children with slightest doubt, as we all know that there is a time-frame for the development of binocular stereoscopic vision.

Reduced stereoacuity can be associated with number of vision affecting disorders including strabismus, amblyopia, and refractive disorders. Stereoacuity testing is, therefore, used clinically for detecting visual disorders and more importantly for monitoring sensory binocularity. Demonstration of normal age-matched stereoacuity indicates normal development of sensory and motor functions.

Stereoscopic vision is not an 'all or none' phenomenon, since the ability to judge relative depth with binocular single vision depends upon and varies with visual acuity, illumination, duration of stimuli, absolute distance, and size of the visual field. Stereocauity, more precisely, is the smallest amount of horizontal retinal image disparity that gives rise to a sensation of relative depth and is expressed as the visual angle in seconds of an arc (an arc is part of a circle), and is measured in minutes present in that arc or seconds in one minute of arc.

Normal adult stereoacuity varies according to different studies between 20 and 40 seconds of arc. On a broader aspect, stereocauity higher than 40 sec/arc is considered abnormal.

When one attempts to apply this standard to paediatric age group, the problem of patient co-operation is compounded by a lack of proper information about the age at which full stereoacuity develops.

In a study where stereoacuity was tested in 300 children, aged 3 to 13 years, data showed gradual improvement in stereo-acuity with increasing age, up to 9 years, with a normal stereoacuity of 40 seconds of arc was consistently found. After that the stereoacuity remained constant. Taking the summation of other similar studies, the average stereoacuity in children is as follows: 3 years—300 sec/arc; 5 years—140 sec/arc; 6 years—80 sec/arc; 7 years—60 sec/arc; and 9 years—40 sec/arc. These normal parameters are important to remember when children are tested for stereoacuity in follow-up of treatment for amblyopia and other vision disorders.

There is still controversy regarding development of stereo-acuity in infants and small children of preverbal age. One study showed stereoacuity developed from 300 sec/arc between 6 months and one year to 30 sec/arc at 5 years of age, with maximum improvement around 2 years of age. But most agree that stereoacuity parallels with normal development of visual acuity and normal binocular vision.

Studies in infants using the Forced Preferential Looking test using modified Teller's cards showed that 1 min/arc stereoacuity could be demonstrated in by 4 months of age. The test was performed at 60 cm using modified Teller card, one having the simple sinusoidal grating and other having 3-D grating.

The measurement of stereopsis is an important component of an ocular assessment in vision testing procedures, as it immensely assists in ruling out micro-strabismus or assessing visual loss in amblyopia and anisometropia.

Therefore, evaluation of stereopsis is mandatory in examination protocol of ocular visual disorders in children particularly strabismus, amblyopia, and refractory errors.

PHYSIOLOGY OF STEREOPSIS

The angle formed by rays of light diverging from a near object and entering the eye is larger than that formed by a distant object. In essence, the part nearer to eyes subtends a larger angle than that subtended from a more distant object. Images of objects may not fall on corresponding points on retina, but still can be fused. This disparity of angles subtended on the two retinas, when processed in the visual cortex, forms the basis of stereo-vision.

We are all aware of the Panum's fusional area, which is an elliptical area, along the horopter, where objects present in that area can be fused. The Panum's area is like a band or corridor, thin at the centre and broader at the periphery (Fig. 14.1). The

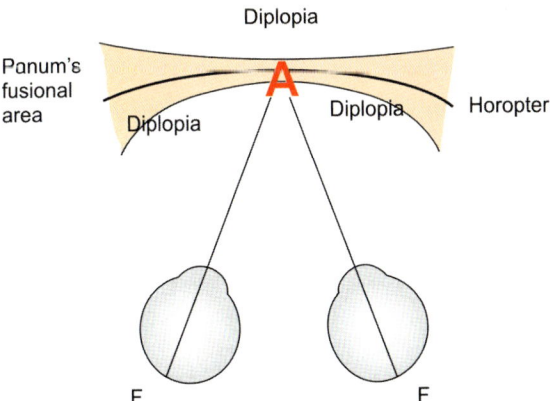

Fig. 14.1: The Panum's fusional area of a person. Beyond this, objects viewed are not fused and produce diplopia.

central part corresponds to the sharpest visual acuity but smaller fusional area; while the periphery has larger fusional capacity.

Stereopsis exists only in the visual cortex where the retinal disparity is processed. Thus, it is a type of hyperacuity. Areas V1 and V2 of visual cortex are the principal areas involved with the processing.

From person-to-person, the ability of stereopsis varies. As a form of hyperacuity, target separation with excellent binocular vision, can be appreciated down to 8–10 sec/arc! But this is not common.

In addition to the above stereoscopic threshold, there are two broad types of stereo-vision. These are often referred to as local and global stereopsis. It is important to know that persons can have local stereopsis in absence of global, but not vice-versa.

It has long been established that global stereopsis appreciation requires association of right occipital cortex neurons and patients with neurological lesions in that area can lose global stereopsis. It has been also found that early onset strabismus in children can result in loss of global stereopsis while local stereopsis may persist.

Global stereopsis means appreciation of stereopsis in the visual field and has implications in children and adults alike. The visual system performs interocular image disparity computations across the binocular visual field. Deficiency of global depth perception causes poor motion detection like assessing relative motions of objects in space, alighting from stairs, moving through crowds, etc. In children, this virtue is important in playing ball games, swimming, etc. Loss of global stereopsis in children reflects fragile fusion and results in intermittent strabismus.

Local stereopsis implies fine stereopsis and judgement of depth perception in static objects, which are relatively near, and limited to the area in vicinity of the target. Local stereopsis is the function of fovea and requires perfect visual acuity.

NEWER CONCEPTS ON STEREO-VISION

The acquisition of binocular vision and stereo-vision was long thought to be impossible unless the person acquired this faculty in infancy or early childhood during a certain 'critical period'. This hypothesis normally went unquestioned and has formed the basis of therapeutic approaches to binocular disorders for decades. But since studies on binocular recovery began to surface in scientific journals, this assumption is now a scientific dogma!

Very recently, there has been a rise in scientific investigations into stereopsis recovery in youths and adults, who had no stereo-vision before. While consensus is developing that an adult 'may' acquire stereo-vision but currently it is not possible to predict as to how much gain may occur. And there is no general agreement on what therapeutic procedure to be applied in these cases.

Most authors summarized the accepted scientific view of the present time as: "Stereopsis will never be obtained unless amblyopia is corrected, the eyes aligned, and binocular fusion achieved before the age of 2 years." But contrary to this notion, there are many exceptions and the exact time-frame cannot be put as a rule, because many crucial pieces of basic science information are still missing.

The general information which is circulated, as a fully accepted medical notion, is: "If an adult has a childhood strabismus that has never been treated, it is too late to 'fully' treat amblyopia and improve stereopsis; and the goal in surgery is simply cosmetic, though sometimes treatment does improve global stereopsis and enlarge side vision."

Recently, however, stereopsis recovery is known to have occurred in number of adults. While this has occurred in some cases after visual exercises or spontaneous visual experiences, the scepticism around non-recovery after certain age is now declining, and strabismus surgery has now become more optimistic with regard to outcome in terms of binocular function and stereopsis. This again brings into light the concept of 'neural plasticity' in adulthood.

TESTS FOR STEREOPSIS

Testing procedures for stereoacuity can be broadly put into three categories:

1. Anaglyphic—requiring use of red-green glasses for dissociation.
2. Vectographic—requiring polarizing glasses.
3. Lenticular—requiring no glasses for viewing 3-D objects.

Titmus fly and related tests are contour-stereograms which measure local stereopsis and have certain monocular clues which may give inaccurate result.

Random dot tests, on the other hand, measure global stereopsis and have almost no monocular clues. Small stereo-targets are likely to be more sensitive for detecting stereo-vision defects than targets of large size.

Each has its own merits and demerits. But some are simple, and are very specific and useful for testing in small children.

Titmus Test or House Fly Test

Titmus test is a vectogram consisting of a polarized stereogram having two polarized images at right angles to each other. When viewed through polarizing filters, it presents one image to one eye and the another to the other eye. When placed on a chart, it becomes a vectograph. The titmus vectogram is a chart based on this principle, in which half of the chart is seen with one eye and the other half by the second eye.

'Titmus' literally means resembling a bird, and the test was developed by Stereo Optical Company, USA, and vectogram is a trademark of this company, which utilizes the principle of polarization in these stereo tests (Fig. 14.2).

The Stereo Optical Co., presents three types of chart in form of a book, viewed from about 40 cm, using polarizing glasses.

The main chart has the house fly. The fly is universally known and understood by very young children. The large central mass and the translucent wings make it an ideal stereoscopic subject. When seen with one eye only, the fly will appear as an ordinary flat photograph. With binocular viewing,

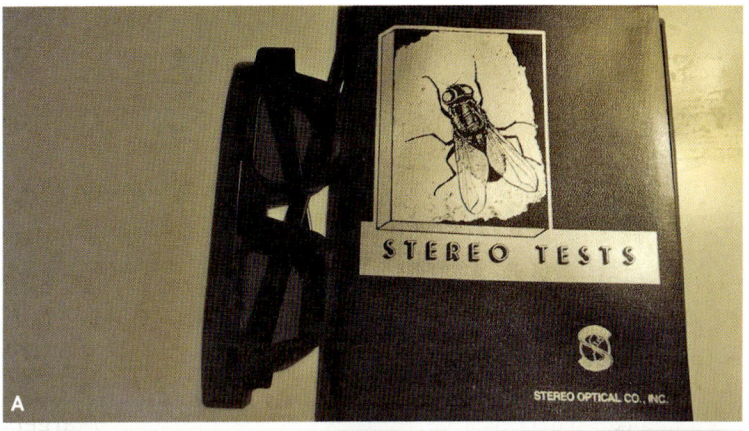

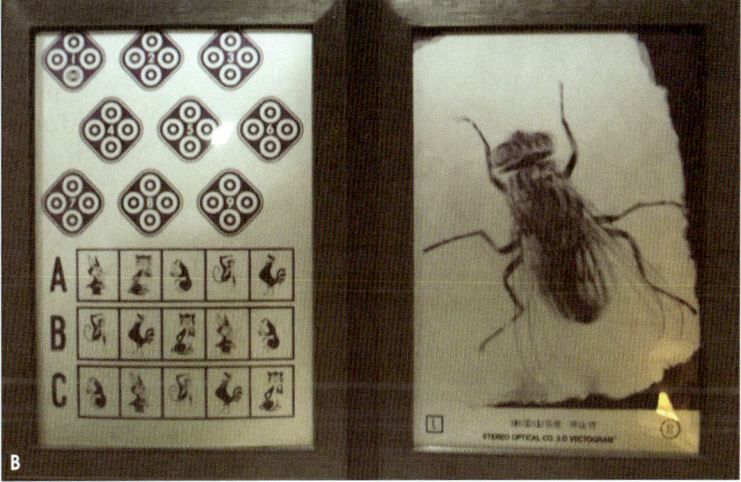

Fig. 14.2A and B: (A) Titmus fly test book by Stereo Optical Company, (B) Titmus fly test and related tests for stereoacuity

the wings will typically appear to come 'out' of the plate. One may ask a child to 'pinch' the wings of the fly, and they will be much above the plate. The book should be held straight in front so as to have the best effect of polarization. One important assumption to be derived is the height at which the child is pinching the wings; if it is too close to the plate, then stereo-acuity is worse. The stereo threshold of the fly test is around 3500 sec/arc or 60 min of arc.

The second plate has two parts: One part has 9 blocks. Each block has 4 circles. One of the circle projects 'out' of the block, when seen with polarizing glasses. The first block has stereo–acuity threshold of 800 sec/arc and the 9th one has 40 sec/arc stereo threshold.

The third part is for more smaller children, having stereoscopic pictures of toys like cat, monkey, squirrel, hen, and rabbit. There are three lines, each having these five pictures, having threshold from 400 sec/arc to 100 sec/arc.

Random-Dot Stereo Tests

All tests based on the principle of random dots was first described by Bela Julesz in 1964.

The TNO Random-Dot Stereo Test (Figs 14.3 and 14.4) was designed by TNO Institute for Perception, Netherland. In this test, the eye sees an array of little characters or dots of uniform texture and containing no recognisable shape or contour. The difference from contour tests is that a certain area has been laterally displaced with respect to the other to produce some retinal disparity. Each plate containing images presented to each eye have been superimposed and printed in colours, and when using red-green filter glasses, they become visible. On

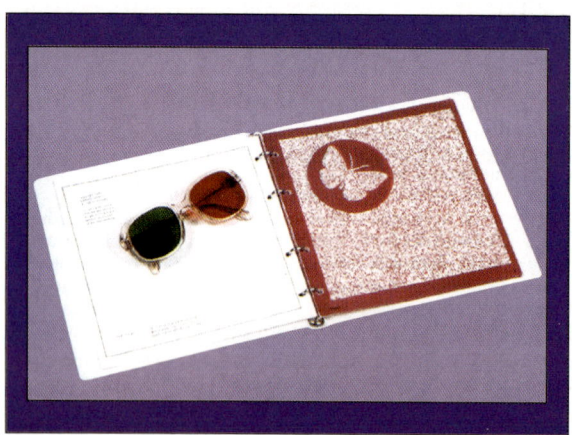

Fig. 14.3: TNO test for stereoacuity

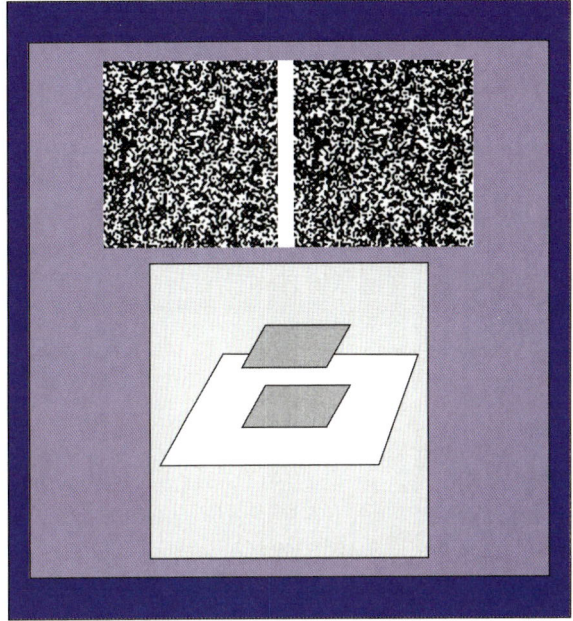

Fig. 14.4: Random-dot test for stereoacuity

its own, neither of the stereo pair is visible but when viewed binocularly, the observer can see a figure either in front or behind the background.

In number of studies in children ranging from 4 to 18 years, the following general consensus has emerged:

a. TNO test is a good screening test for amblyopes where visual acuity cannot be ascertained properly and amblyopia suspects.

b. The red-green anaglyphs used do not pose problems for colour defective children.

c. A stereoacuity of <120 sec/arc is a good predictor of normal or near normal vision; and therefore, may help in evaluating the often incomplete results of vision tests in young children.

The test contains no monocular clues and is excellent test for stereoacuity assessment in amblyopia, suppression and strabismus in children.

Randot Stereo Test

The Randot stereo test is a patent of Stereo Optical Company, and is a 3-D vectogram of plates or sheet. The plates are to be viewed from a distance of 3 metres (10 feet) using polarizing glasses. The test can measure stereoacuity up to 20 sec/arc.

The Randot–E Test: It uses polarized random pattern and requires the use of polarizing glasses to view the object. The subject will see a raised letter 'E' coming out of the surroundings. At 50 cm viewing distance, the stereoscopic effect of E is 500 sec/arc.

Dynamic Random-Dot Test: Recent studies have shown that none of the available stereo tests are very reliable to assess stereoacuity in early amblyopes. Innovative technology has assisted in devising a test known as *moving dynamic Random–Dot stereo test* (MDRS), which is a computer-generated stereo test that uses dynamic random-dot background to minimize false clues, and use of a disparate target that moves horizontally across the screen in a random fashion. Dissociation is by red-

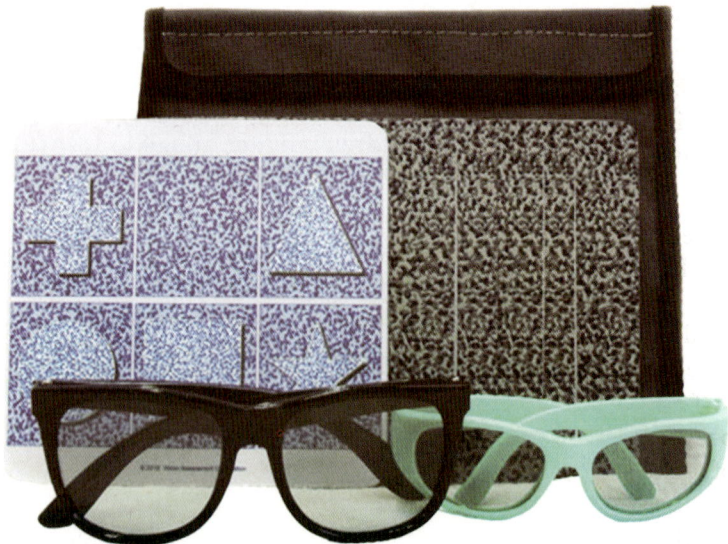

Fig. 14.5: Random-dot test with polaroid glasses for children

green filter glasses. The test was developed to measure stereo thresholds in infants, small children and multiple handicaps.

The test is quite similar to Forced Preferential Looking method and has showed promise in testing infants to 6 years of age and reliability that 75% times the response is positive.

MDRS test has been shown to be sensitive measure of visual development, demonstrating visual performance in sense of stereoacuity and proving that it is still developing up to age of 9 years.

As MDRS is a high-order test requiring good performance of visual functions to pass it, but studies have demonstrated that the test shows promise for being sensitive for detection of anisometropia and strabismic amblyopia.

Lang Test

Lang's test was designed to simplify stereo-vision in children. It is based on two principles, i.e. random dots and cylindrical gratings. The test is a single card held by the examiner at 50 cm. It has 3 levels of stereo threshold, all at low levels. The Lang stereo test was developed by Swiss ophthalmologist Joseph Lang in 1980s. This easy-to-use test is applied for early detection of visual problems in infants and children. The test is becoming very popular owing to its simplicity and ease of administration by general ophthalmologists and paediatricians as well (Fig. 14.6).

Two versions are available: The Lang stereo tests I and II, which differ only in the type of objects to be recognised. The Lang test II additionally contains a picture that can be seen with one eye, i.e. a star. The test plates are solid and thick, and can be easily carried around. These can be put into a fitting carrying case, with a instruction manual.

The Lang stereo-pad is a new system, using the same principle. It has been created to compliment the main function of stereopsis using the preferential looking procedure.

Since the test had been primarily developed for children, the three objects chosen are quite common to recognise at this age. The three objects in Lang I test are a cat, a star, and a car.

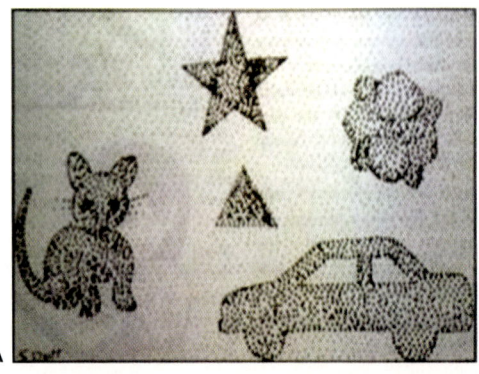

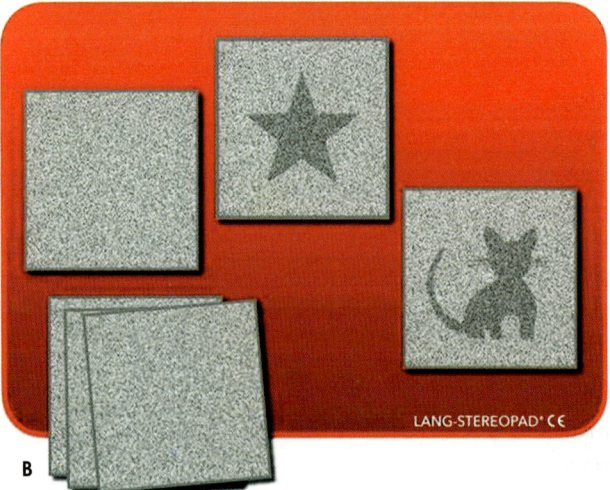

Fig. 14.6A and B: Lang stereo test

Lang II test contains an elephant, a car and half-moon. The most prominent object is the cat (1200 sec/arc), the elephant (600 sec/arc), and the star (1000 sec/arc). The Lang StereoPad has 6 objects of varying disparity, i.e. star (1000); car (600); cat (400); moon (200); and sun (100 sec/arc), respectively.

Frisby Davis Test

Frisby Davis (FD2) Test is the most useful subjective stereo test for infants and children. It is simple and easy-to-administer,

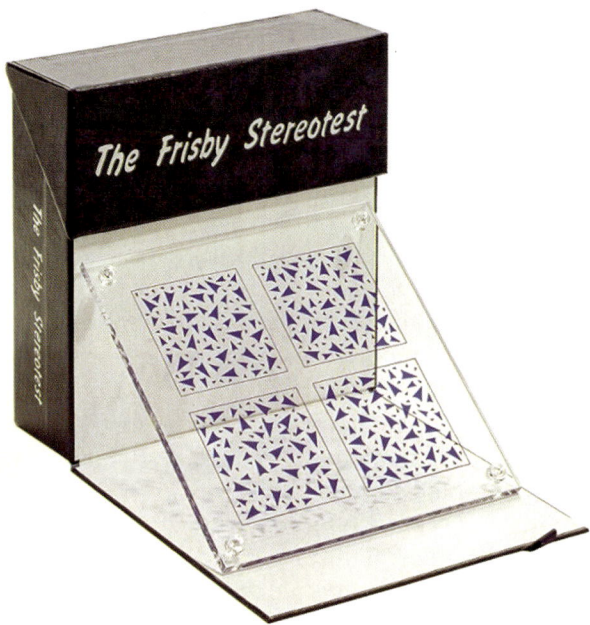

Fig. 14.7: Frisby Davis stereotest

no need for any special glasses, and good for amblyopia assessment (Fig. 14.7).

Stereoacuity testing by this method showed distance stereoacuity reaches adult levels by approximately 5 years of age, which is much early as compared to other test results. Nevertheless, it is certain that abnormal values after this age should be taken with caution.

The test presented at 40 cm the patient has to locate the arc of the moon (200 sec arc), a star (200 sec arc), a car (400 sec arc) and an elephant (600 sec arc).

Frisby Davis is available for both distance and near stereo testing. The near test is more applicable for children and consists of a book with three plates. Each plate has four random pattern squares. In one of the squares is embedded a target, usually a circle. An observer with normal binocular stereo-vision will be able to see the target lying in-depth relative to its surroundings.

The thickness of the plate also varies. The thickest plate having more in-depth target and more easily seen. The thinner the plate and greater the distance, the better the stereoacuity.

A large study was done with Frisby test on population ranging from children to older persons, with testing distance from 1 to 6 metres. The results were analysed in three groups: 'visually developing', aged 3 to 9 years; 'visually mature', aged 10 to 50 years; and 'older' aged 50 to 80 years. The stereoacuity levels was 25, 20 and 85 sec/arc, respectively. This test is also useful in monitoring the visual status in intermittent exotropia. Stereoacuity going below the age matched stereocauity in children is an indication for surgical intervention.

As with the fly test, the child has to be instructed what is expected from him. First, present the thickest plate and observe the reaction. Infants will often spontaneously touch the target-in-depth. If this does not happen, draw attention by pointing one of the child's finger at the target. Now take the plate further away and place it upside down or tilt it to a new position and present it afresh. And again ask the child to point at the target. Repeat this procedure with thinner plates, until the end point is achieved. With Frisby test, it is feasible to test stereoacuity <1 year of age.

Bernell Stereo Reindeer Test

The test is marketed by Bernell Corporation and is similar to titmus fly test, using polarizing glasses for detecting the object. The object instead of fly is a reindeer, which is well known in western world and familiar to children. One specificity which stands out is that the nose of reindeer can be made to wiggle by rotating the picture slightly, which makes the test more attractive to children. In some plates, a reindeer is replaced by a dinosaur (Fig. 14.8).

BINOCULAR TRAINING

It is universally agreed that the earlier the treatment of aniso-metropia, amblyopia, and strabismus, the better the chances of regaining binocular vision and stereopsis. Most of the times, with successful treatment of the above conditions, as the visual

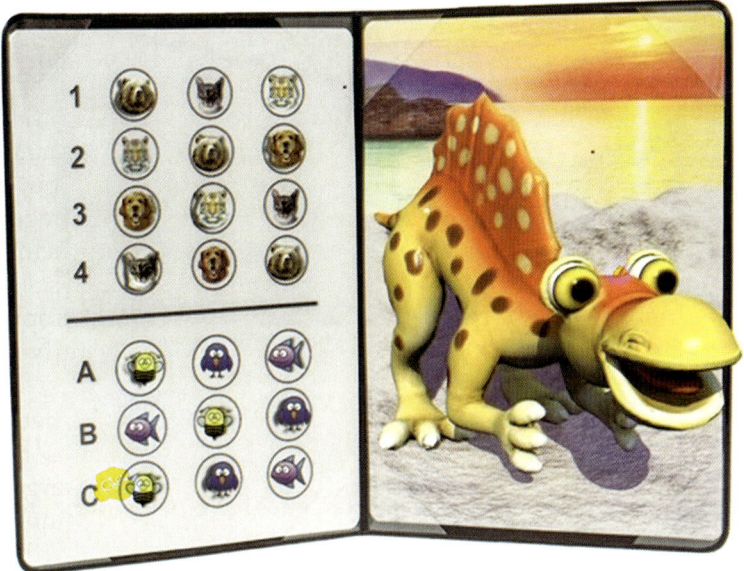

Fig. 14.8: Bernell stereo test for small children

acuity improves, so occurs spontaneous improvement in stereopsis. Let us see some reports.

In a study of 45 adults over 18 years of age, who underwent surgical correction after having lived with strabismus all along with no surgical intervention or orthoptic training, with visual acuity of 6/12 to 6/18 in the deviated eye, stereopsis was present in 80% of exotropes and 30% of esotropes. In another study, 36 patients aged 8 to 30 years with long-standing exotropia since early childhood and had preoperative stereopsis of 400 sec/arc or less regained spontaneously binocular vision and stereopsis of 200 sec/arc after surgical intervention.

In contrast, in a group of 20 adults, all of whom received surgical correction for long-standing untreated esotropia, showed binocular fusion and an increased visual field but none demonstrated any improvement in stereo-vision one year postoperatively.

These are some of the examples of postoperative results on status of stereo-vision. There is still controversy whether any orthoptic or other type of any modern therapy would be bene-

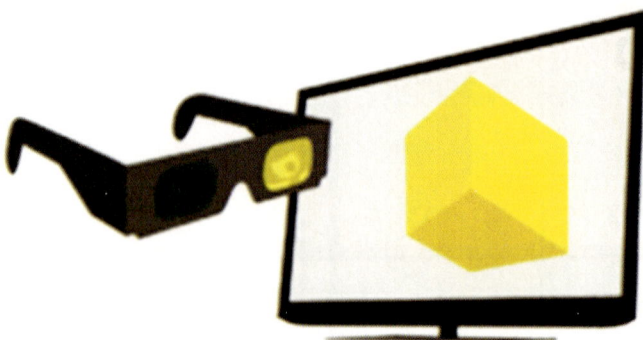

Fig. 14.9: 3-D shutter glasses

ficial in improving stereopsis later in life or even in children, post-treatment of amblyopia and strabismus.

Lately, so-called 'binocular exercises' have been in practice for improving binocular fusion and stereopsis and are known as 'dicoptic or binocular training'. Some examples are as follows:

1. *3-D Shutter Glasses:* Shutter glasses are a pair of polarized lenses with a coating of liquid crystal on the glass. It works by only presenting the image intended for left eye while blocking the right eye view; then presenting the right eye image to right eye while blocking the left eye image. The alternate blocking system is due to voltage passed into the liquid crystal layer. The process is so rapid that interruptions do not interfere with the perceived fusion of the two images into a single 3-D image (Fig. 14.9).

2. *Tetris Vedeo Game:* A special video game developed at McGill University showed that one to three weeks of playing a dichoptic video game for 1–2 hours daily can improve stereoacuity. No data was provided.

3. *Similar dichoptic* (use of two eye simultaneously) video games have been developed by University of Rochester, USA, which are called 'virtual reality computer games' to strengthen stereopsis. Since these are not commercially available, detailed discussion will not be put here.

Peripheral Vision

Peripheral vision or the field of vision is the extent and sensitivity of a person's peripheral vision.

Sensitivity of visual field pertains to the quality of peripheral vision, i.e. whether the objects in the visual field are clear or blurred. Field loss can be absolute (no objects seen) or relative (small or dim objects not seen).

The 'field of vision' is that portion of space in which objects are visible at the same moment of steady central fixation. The monocular visual field consists of central vision, and the peripheral vision which in normal adults extends 100° laterally, 60° superiorly and medially, and 70° inferiorly. A vertical line bisects central fixation and divides the visual field into nasal and temporal halves. Situated in the temporal half is the 'blind spot' approximately 12° to 17° from the fixation and 1.5° below the horizontal meridian. The blind spot corresponds to the optic disc and is represented on the chart as an 'absolute scotoma'.

In children, the normal visual field is similar to adults after 5 years of age. Before this age, the figures are not known in literature; though 'confrontation' tests have been tried but they are tentative with unreliable results. Further, the fields so obtained are slightly less than adult norms. Most reliable and reproducible results have been obtained above 9 years of age.

The size and quality of visual fields are important basic functions to be assessed as part of functional visual assessment. This becomes far more important when visual assessment is done in children with retinal or central nervous system anomalies.

A review of literature indicates stark disagreement on the rate of peripheral vision development in children and age of peripheral visual maturation.

Normal maturation of peripheral vision has been reported as early as 5 years of age and as later as 13 years. These vast maturation differences result from hugely different methods of testing. For example, use of static versus kinetic stimuli makes a difference as well as stimulus velocity and intensity also vary considerably. Stimulus used in adults may not conform to the testing in children. Furthermore, the age, mental status, cognitive development, co-operation, testing conditions, reproducibility, the type of test used, and expertise of the technician, etc. all change the reliability of results.

Therefore, assessment expectations are needed for specific way of testing and use of instruments. The only study to-date to report 'reaction time' (RT) in children on semikinetic perimetry (SKP) on Octopus perimeter is by Vonthein et al. They tested children between 10 and 18 years of age, and found no difference between this group and 20–60 years group. Normative values using SKP on Octopus for children above 9 years are limited and below this age are unknown. Normative data for blind spot area are also not documented in children. Use of Goldmann perimeter has not proved successful in children and hence is not used.

A recent study examined normative blind spot size using SKP using 3 stimulus luminosities all at 2°/second speed, on Octopus. The blind spot scotoma was found to decrease with increased luminous intensity and measurements were most repeatable. Blind spot size with SKP testing in children has not been previously reported, neither is known how potential optic nerve and fixation stability may affect apparent blind spot size with age.

The important fact is that the ability to accurately plot the blind spot scotoma is often clinically recorded as measure of reliability of field testing. Dolderer et al in 2006 reported the minimum size of blind spot to be 17°. The expected age at which the blind spot can be accurately measured in children is not confirmed.

Static perimetry strategies are false positive, false negative, and fixation loss indices are higher. Large variations in reaction time (RT) are found in children and their reliability in static perimetry are unknown or unsuitable as RT to visual stimuli gradually reduces between ages 4 and 11 years, and is slower than adults.

A number of practical aspects need to be considered when testing visual fields in children. A number of recommendations have been provided by some authors for successful testing on perimetry such as use of a cushion, continuous monitoring of fixation and head position, verbal assurances, reminders to blink, and informing the child of test progress. Also it is advisable to prime the child with a 'practice stimuli', prior to actual testing, to ensure they understood the test.

Semikinetic perimetry using the Octopus perimeter is becoming the test of choice in children by many clinicians due to more standardized method compared to Goldmann perimeter and good retest reliability. Despite this, there are limited normative published data of visual fields, reaction time, and blind spot size as a function of age. One of the largest and clinically reliable study was done by Anne Bjerre et al as late as 2014 on more than 200 children aged between 5 and 17 years using the Octopus-900 perimeter. Their results showed that reliability of visual fields (VF) markedly increases by 11–12 years of age. After 12 years of age, adult-like performance persists on all reliability measures. The only other study has examined automatic kinetic perimetry in children from age 5 to 12 years, using the Twinfield perimeter. The results were similar to the study done by Bjerre et al.

Using automatic 'static perimetry' on 28 children, Wabbels and Wilscher reported that reliable results and ability to fully complete the testing strategies could be obtained in all children at age 13 years.

Blumenthal et al using 'frequency-doubling' perimetry showed only 47% reliability in children younger than 8 years, and 75% reliability in children older than 8 years. On the other hand, Morales and Brown had performed automated static perimetry with Octopus in 50 normal children and showed that reliable, consistent results can be obtained in children at 7 years age.

There is controversy in the literature regarding developmental change in VF area. Studies using automatic kinetic perimetry found no change with age; while manual kinetic perimetry using Goldmann perimeter showed a developmental increase in the field area after 5 years of age.

The ultimate inference from all above studies is that below 5 years of age reliability in results is doubtful and we do not have reliable normative data of children below that age. Therefore, visual field test results should be guarded in interpretations, and expressed only after taking all safeguards and recommendations into consideration. Also the clinical aspect should be strongly correlated with the results.

Another important point is that in infants below 6 months of age, any type of field testing by any means, such as 'confrontation' method, should not be attempted owing to their instability of eye movements. Above 6 months of age, qualitative field assessment has been tried using the 'forced preferential looking' testing method using the Teller's cards. The eye 'fixation' movements have been taken as a measure of field when the card is brought from periphery to the centre of vision.

An attempt had been made to assess fields in children between 2 and 5 years of age using a 'light-emitting diode (LED) perimeter'. The results have been compared in same group of children using Goldmann perimeter. The results have been found to be similar to children above 9 years of age, but the reproducibility lacked tremendously and hence is not quoted for reference.

IMPLICATIONS OF FIELD LOSS IN CHILDREN

A complete right or left visual field loss (hemianopia) may affect scanning eye movements so crucial in reading or writing that it can make near work difficult and inefficient. Reading will be more difficult for a child with right field hemianopia, as we make small, saccadic eye movements to the right as we read a line from left to right. In complete right field loss, there is no vision to the right of fixation and thus no decoding cue process. But children may learn to read with repeated right–left saccades in order to read the text. Using a finger to scroll along the line or text may be helpful in reading.

In children with left-sided hemianopia, the problem involves returning from right end of line to left which makes reading extremely difficult and may cause confusion in understanding the written text.

Inferior field loss affects scanning downwards and poses a bigger handicap. The solution for such handicaps is to move the whole written material upwards rather than move the eyes downwards.

For a child, with any type of field loss, it is important to ensure that the child is aware of the handicap and made to scrutinize the text as a whole.

Children with major field losses may neglect or ignore to read and wright or draw on the part of the sheet that falls into their non-seeing part.

Solutions for these defects may be as follows:

- Keep the paper slanted for inferior or superior field loss.
- Lined paper may be used.
- The child should be taught to use the entire paper sheet. This is done by prior showing the whole picture or written material to him/her.

Children with field loss often develop head tilt or turn to aid in scanning the non-seeing part. Consistent such manoeuvres indicate child's self-created adaptation to their field loss. This point should always be kept in mind while evaluating reasons for head tilt or turn.

Another important innovative move is to place the child in the classroom in such a way that the child sees the whole class and teacher. For example, a child with 'right field loss' should be seated to the right side of the class; while a child with 'left field loss' should be seated on the left side of the class.

Mobility is another issue with children with major field losses. Safety during movement is a very important consideration and appropriate precautions should be observed while moving in public or playing games. Absolute or complete hemifield loss is detrimental to safe mobility and children with such defects will have difficulty in localising objects or recognising people, even if their visual acuity is normal!

It is strongly recommended that a child with such hemianopic field defects should be trained for comprehensive orientation of body and spatial concepts, safety measures while travelling, walking, visual scanning skills, and ability to judge distance and depth. Such training has to be imparted in specially trained centres or by trained personnel who are adept in training of visually handicapped persons.

We learn to use information for orientation in environment only if we actively participate in movement and recognition. A study was done by Dr. Lea Hyverinen on a child who had large left hemianopic defect. Such monocular defects usually occur in cortical lesions in areas responsible for spatial awareness and planning. The child was repeatedly shown videos of his route from school to home and back, which he memorized and this lead to his independent movement from school and back. Such training is an essential part of rehabilitation for such defects. Lower field loss effectively disturbs mobility. The child walks with head bent down to compensate for his disability. Some children can get along using strong prism glasses. The effects on reading also depends upon the size of macular sparing. If there is no macular sparing, then a right-sided hemianopia makes saccades to right letter inadequate and thus the child tilts his head to the right or tilts the page to view the text.

FUNCTIONAL FIELD LOSSES

Before we embark on the specificities of field losses, it would be not out of place to understand a few basic concepts.

1. **Anterior visual pathways** include the two eyes and the pathway up to the lateral geniculate nucleus (LGN), i.e. before the visual pathway enters the substance of the brain.

2. **Posterior visual pathways** include fibres from LGN to the primary visual cortical areas.

Another fact (explained elsewhere in the book) is that the 'central parts of the visual field' occupy much larger 'visual cortical area' in relation to the peripheral parts of visual field, and are magnified known as 'cortical magnification'. That is why, we see details of centrally placed objects more vividly than objects in the peripheral field. Almost half of the visual cortex is represented by central 12°–13° of visual field.

Visual system has another basic property, i.e. visual information that is 'not moving', loses its representation in a few seconds (Fig. 15.1).

In Fig. 15.1, focus your sight at the 'stop' sign. Initially, the dark area at the upper right corner will be visible; but after a few seconds, it will start disappearing from sight.

This phenomenon is important when assessing scotomas. Areas of visual field where nothing is happening disappear from consciousness! Every one of us has a blind spot—corresponding to the nerve head—yet we cannot see it, though it can be demonstrated on perimetry. That is why kinetic perimetry is now becoming more useful than static perimetry, especially in children. If the stimulus in static method is kept for a longer time, children very quickly lose interest and it disappears from sight.

Scotomas caused by retinal changes are subjectively experienced when they are large. In the very centre of visual field,

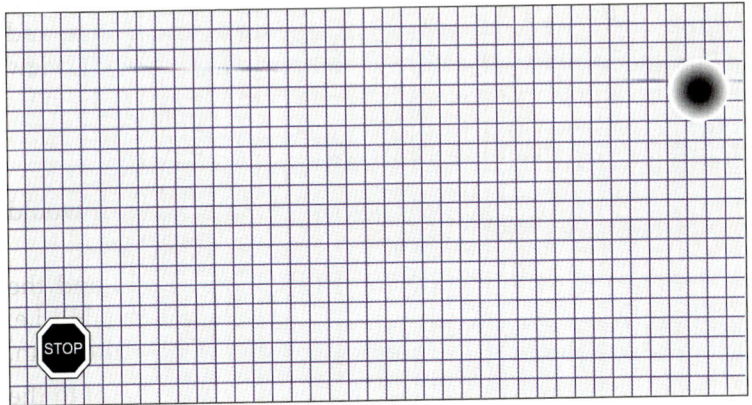

Fig. 15.1: Chart depicting disappearance of static scotoma at right upper quadrant

the subjective experience of a scotoma depends upon the type of lesion causing it. If there is bleeding on or into the retina, there is a dark shadow in the subjective field. If the bleeding is behind the retina, the scotoma appears as a hazy area in the corresponding field of vision. So when we assess the recordings of perimetry, we should not take them on face value, but should ask the patient what he/she subjectively experiences.

Scotomas caused by damage to the posterior visual pathways may be only partial because visual information has been already transferred via the tectal pathways to the cortical visual areas. In this scenario, magnocellular information dominates and thus 'movement perception' may be present even if form perception is completely lost. Unfortunately, 'movement perception' is not assessed as part of clinical examinations. Also, assessment of 'colour perception', which is equally important, is forgotten. It is, therefore, important that while assessing fields in suspected damage to visual pathways, colour and motion should also be examined.

There is one more physiologic function that we need to be aware of when examining functional visual field, i.e. short-term memory and sensorium. Since the eye moves, the area of scotoma falls on different objects in the environment and visual information from adjacent areas fills in the area of scotoma and thus a small scotoma does not have any functional significance. Even large scotomas can be effectively filled in by visual information stored in the short-term memory (visual memory).

Another problem in assessing scotomas induced by lesions in the posterior visual areas is loss of 'sensorium'. Subjective information assessed for such lesions cannot be relied upon due to incoherent behaviour which appear in brain lesions.

ORGANIZATION OF FIELD LOSSES

A brief account of description of field defects is as follows:
1. Major field loss
2. Minor field loss
3. Distortion of image
4. Perceptual loss without measurable field loss
5. Restriction of visual field due to motor problems.

Major Field Loss

Comprises of loss of one-half of visual field (hemianopias), central loss of field, or total loss of field.

Total field defects occur in lesions of the eye itself or the anterior visual pathways. Usually one or both eyes may be involved. Some of causes in eye comprise of retinitis of prematurity, retinitis pigmentosa, colobomas, congenital glaucoma, retinal detachment (inflammatory or traumatic), etc.

Total loss of field in one eye occurs in lesions of anterior pathways before optic chiasma like trauma, orbital tumours, inflammatory conditions, vascular lesions, etc.

Central loss of field usually consists of loss of central 10–12° and is usually caused by maculopathies, congenital or acquired.

Hemianopias are commonly found in lesions around optic chiasma or optic tract.

Field Loss due to Disorders of Eye

The most common causes of field loss in children are ROP, congenital glaucoma, colobomas, and retinitis pigmentosa. ROP and congenital glaucoma lead to constriction of the visual field. There may be several scotomas inside the visual field or the 'sensitivity 'of the whole field may be reduced. These changes cause difficulty in orientation and mobility. In colobomas, since there is no retina in the lower part, the corresponding upper field is totally missing. The lesion may involve one or both eyes. When in both eyes, the blind areas are seldom symmetrical.

Retinitis pigmentosa has several variants, with different speeds of development and variations in field defects. The most common type starts in the 'mid-periphery'. This area corresponds to the maximum concentration of rod cells in the retina. Initially, there may be patchy field loss. By and by, these patches enlarge and combine to form partial or complete ring scotoma. Although this so-called ring scotoma may not show response to the largest, brightest stimuli on Goldmann perimeter but might show perception of flicker and movement. Children with ring scotomas do not have difficulty in mobility or reading.

Central Scotomas

Central scotomas damage the very centre of visual field. There may remain some minute areas of vision within the scotoma. The child learns to use the best area of visual quality available and thus develops an 'extrafoveal fixation' at this 'preferred retinal locus' (PRL). If the locus with best resolution is very small, the child may use another retinal area with relatively less retinal acuity but larger viewing area. In assessing the reading or near field, it is interesting to know whether the child uses different fixation areas. This is done by an 'extrafoveal fixation recorder.'

Extrafoveal fixation recorder: The quality of central field is important to access for sustained near visual tasks like reading and writing. In these tasks, small visual scotomas, areas of diminished sensitivity, and distortions of images can disturb the visual task.

In routine clinical work, scotomas are mapped using perimeters. They are large and expensive. A simple campimeter developed by Dr. Bertil Damato is useful for mapping central visual field. In this, stimulus appears in the middle of a test screen while the subject looks at numbers placed at different locations on the screen. The untested eye is covered. A pointer with a ring at its end is placed on the number to help the child maintain fixation on it. It is wise to start with a few points at the centre and then measure the blind spot. If the blind spot can be located and mapped, other central scotomas can also be detected. If the child has a central scotoma and fixation has shifted to other 'preferred retinal location' (PRL), the blind spot will also be shifted in the same direction and the child will have a visual response when a stimulus is shown in the area of normal blind spot. If the child does not fixate with fovea, the whole visual map will be shifted in the direction opposite to the PRL, i.e. if the new fixation area is above the central lesion, the shadow of the lesion will be located above the area of fixation and the blind spot will be shifted up.

Minor Field Loss

Small lesions in the retina may cause minor visual field defects usually occurring after trauma with organized haemorrhage in the retina or defunct area after repair of a retinal detachment. Usually, such small areas are not subjectively observed as they are compensated from the other eye visual field. Small damage to the optic tract or chiasma or optic radiation will appear on perimetry when specifically tested for suspected brain damage. Since small field defects are common in children with even mild forms of periventricular leucomalacia, CVI may result and reading should be tested and taught using different text sizes to become aware of the quality of reading field of the child.

Distortion of Image

Distortion of image occurs commonly due to multiple, close, small scotomas occurring due to stretching or folds in the retina. When present from early childhood they are difficult to diagnose as the child is so accustomed to the image quality that they seldom complain about the contour of things around them. Older children may complain subjective defect in image quality when compared with narration by other normal children. Different magnifications can be used to correct the defect, if not treatable.

Perceptual Losses without Measurable Field Loss

Preceptual losses do not belong to assessment of visual field. They are mentioned here as they sometimes mimic a visual scotoma. A typical situation is loss of recognition of facial features. The child has normal visual acuity and sees minute details but does not recognise family members by face. In such situations, distortion of image of central scotoma may be suspected. However, the visual fields show normal pattern. Such cases of 'visual agnosia' commonly occur after brain haemorrhage, head trauma, or in CVI (cortical visual impairments.)

Restriction of Functional Visual Field due to Motor Problems

Functional visual field is much larger than the binocular visual field. Because the eyes move, we are aware of some 20°–30° extra visual field behind us. If the movement of eyes is restricted and need to be compensated with head movements—which ought to be learned—the field becomes smaller than normal. Spastic children with uncontrolled head and body movements cannot use their full potential of visual field. Often motor disturbance in intraocular muscles also occurs simultaneously in these children, causing transient myopia and creating visual blur.

Visually impaired children may have visual defects of many different kinds. Clinical measurements often give a good start to the functional assessment but should not be taken as complete and true description of the visual field. For orientation in the environment, true assessment of the fields, scotomas, and training to overcome the field defect are important.

TESTING OF FIELD DEFECTS

Visual field (VF) testing is key parameter in assessing and monitoring visual function in patients with ophthalmic and neurological diseases.

We do not have any data on the number of children in India undergoing perimetry tests but western countries like UK or USA almost 3000–3500 children under age 16 undergo formal perimetry every year. There is also paucity of solid data on the correct interpretation of these tests, particularly on reliability in younger children. Number of studies worldwide have at least confirmed one view that perimetry under 5 years of age is not reliable. Also till date, only a few studies are available who have investigated perimetry in normal children. Furthermore, variation in findings relating to test feasibility and reliability have put a question mark on testing strategies.

In general, Humphrey (SITA algorithm) and Goldmann perimetry are the two most commonly utilized in clinical practice in children. Prior studies have tested feasibility of

Goldmann perimetry with single isopters with large stimuli (V4e and III4e) along limited test meridians, limiting their ability to give complete information.

Semiautomated kinetic perimetry (Octopus 900) is reported to be feasible in children, but there is no evidence regarding its comparative feasibility and reliability which is necessary to understand whether this can replace Goldmann perimeter as the perimeter of choice in children.

Assessment of reliability with static perimetry currently relies on the use of automated indices like false positive, false negative, fixation losses, etc. In adults, results and reproducibility has not been associated with these indices and, therefore, assessment of reliability and subsequent interpretation of results in children using static perimetry is currently unknown.

In a recent, well-documented study in children aged between 5 and 15 years was done by Cumberland and Patel in 2015 assessing feasibility, reliability and repeatability of visual fields using all three commonly used Humphrey static, Goldmann and Octopus kinetic perimetry. The results showed overall feasibility by Goldmann as 96.0%; Octopus-900 as 89.0% and Humphrey static was 100%. As for reliability, it was rated as 81.0% for Goldmann; 64.05% for Octopus and 63.0% for Humphrey. Reliability improved with increasing age. Thus, Goldmann perimetry was the most reliable method in children under 15 years of age. The above researchers have surmized that quality perimetry is possible in children as young as 5 years, although the prospects of reliability improve with age. After 9 years of age, all the currently available perimetry tests are reliable. Currently, there are no standardized methods for scoring test reliability in kinetic perimetry.

We know that there are a number of handicaps for reliable performance for perimetry in children. Fatigue is known to impact on test reliability and outcomes. For static perimetry, this affects the accuracy of entire test, whereas points plotted by kinetic perimetry are more reliable as by default, a child still remains attentive on moving objects.

Thus, for children who tire quickly or struggle with extended testing, a quick but reasonably informative test algorithm has to be devised. In such cases, a baseline 'kinetic test' can give valuable information on visual field sensitivity that cannot be achieved by static perimetry techniques.

A balance has to be found between performing the test quickly without jeopardizing the results. It should also be ensured that the child does not feel overwhelmed by the test and is comfortable and attentive.

A preview of the test should be given and the test should be well explained. Another point to be kept in mind is that the test should be performed by the clinician himself, who is well versed with the test and is a bonafide paediatric ophthalmologist who understands the child psychology and knows the handling of children.

One caution to remember is testing of children with delayed milestones or behavioural problems. A 'behavioural visual field test' (BVFT) is a screening test developed specifically for use in such children. A large, longitudinal, retrospective study showed that a population of children with VF defects show changes in sensitivity that are presumed to be learning/developmental defects.

Though visual field tests are a valuable diagnostic tool but are only one facet of a clinical examination and care should be taken not to over/under value individual test results. Formal perimetry should be attempted in children with suspected visual field loss but the type of test and age should be taken into consideration.

For those children where formal perimetry is not possible due to any reason, child specific novel methods have been suggested. These consist of suprathreshold tests using eye-tracking or using certain modified perimeters. Other techniques use game-based or behavioural engagements. These allow for some degree of quantification but need specialized equipment and trained personnel. Goldmann, Humphery and Octopus-900 perimetry are highly feasible in children, with Goldmann perimetry being the most reliable under 9 years of age. Above this age, all methods are equally reliable and normative, age appropriate data exist for each perimetry technique. Thus, the choice of perimetry method rests on the tester regarding age of the child and the clinical condition.

Another study done by Bjerre et al. and published in Neuro-ophthalmology Journal in 2014, assessed the normative field area, feasibility and repeatability using semi-automated kinetic perimetry (Octopus-900) in children ranging from 5 years to young adults up to 22 years. They assessed with 14e and 12e stimulus at 5°/sec and 3°/sec speed. Out of 221 healthy and normal individuals tested, 98% of older children (13 to 22 years) gave reliable results. Reliability decreased with early age as reliability rate was 64% in children between 9 and 12 years and only 24% between 5 and 12 years of age. Blind spot presentation remained unchanged throughout all ages above 5 years. Visual field areas remained unchanged using 5°/sec. speed but increased with 3°/sec. speed, indicating stimulus could be easily followed at slower speeds.

In small children or who are mentally compromised, equipment-based testing may not be feasible. In such children, a simple, conventional 'confrontation technique' is usually helpful.

Confrontation Method

Confrontation field testing is simple but it is essential to master the technique and should not be taken casually. The following steps are a useful guide:

1. Ask the child to look at your nose, or show your fingers briefly in area of central fixation. Each eye is tested individually.

2. Move and flash fingers from periphery to centre making sure that the eye is fixed at your nose. It is best to flash one or two fingers as a target; too many fingers may be confusing.

3. To depict 'double simultaneous perception', flash fingers of both hands in nasal and temporal hemifields. Again the child should maintain fixation.

A number of permutation-combination may be tried. For instance, with patients right eye fixing, show one finger with left hand in temporal field and two fingers with right hand in nasal field. Then show two fingers with left hand and one finger with right hand. If the child sees only one finger in first case and in second part sees two fingers only, then a nasal field defect of right eye is suspected.

Hold both hands in the hemifield under suspicion (e.g. right nasal field loss) and flash fingers above and below the horizontal meridian thereby testing the upper and lower limits of affected hemifield.

In case the child is not able to fixate on the nose (though the human face is an excellent fixation target) alternatively, an interesting fixation target may be brought into central fixation—which is one of our most primitive visual reflexes.

Colour perception is more refined and more sensitive parameter of visual field function. A relative lack of colour perception in one-half of field may be the salient manifestation of an active or resolved intracranial lesion. Therefore, use of a brightly coloured target for testing visual fields is a more appropriate target.

A comparison of brightness or richness of colour can also be used to assess nasal versus temporal field defects. Each eye is tested individually. To explore possibility of subtle hemianopic defects, two similarly coloured objects are held before the patient with one in the nasal and other in the temporal field of vision. The patient, while maintaining central fixation, tells whether the two objects appear similar or either of the two appears dull or brighter. Appearance of dullness arises suspicion of a subtle field defect and should be further explored. In suspected cases, the coloured object should always be moved from dull area to brighter zone and the line of demarcation should be carefully noted to understand the zone of field defect, i.e. quandrantic or an island of defect or even a centrocecal defect.

LOCALIZATION OF FIELD DEFECTS

It would be wise to briefly understand certain visual field defects and source of origin.

The retina is a well-differentiated, stratified sensory membrane. Incident light eventually stimulates the ganglion cell layer and axons from this cellular layer course towards the optic disc in three basic patterns:

1. A papillomacular bundle, which arises from macula and surrounding central retina
2. Superior and inferior arcuate bundles which come from temporal retina
3. Radial bundles from the nasal retina.

The papillomacular bundle from the central 30° of retina represent almost 90% of all retinal fibres in the optic nerve. Lesions in the papillomacular bundle produce central or centrocecal scotomas.

The arcuate fibres surround the papillomacular bundle arising from above, below and temporal to it. Lesions of the arcuate bundles produce arcuate or 'cuneate-shaped' scotomas.

Damage to the superior arcuate bundle for instance in glaucoma manifests as inferior arcuate scotoma and *vice-versa*.

Lesions of nasal retinal axons produce temporal field defects. If nasal fibres nearest to macula are spared, the resulting field defect shows sparing of paramacular temporal field. But if the nasal fibre component of papillomacular fibres and radial fibres are involved, a temporal hemianopic defect results.

Optic Chiasma

All the nasal fibres decussate in the optic chiasma but the inferior nasal fibres first turn rostrally into the opposite optic nerve before projecting back into the opposite optic tract. This anterior elbow of the inferior nasal fibres into the opposite optic nerve is called the 'Wilbrand's knee'. Lesions of the posterior optic nerve before joining the optic chiasma (Wilbrand's area) will produce ipsilateral vision defect and an upper temporal field defect in the contralateral eye.

Damage to the body of the optic chiasma itself produces 'bitemporal hemianopia', usually incongruous.

Optic Tract

Lesions of the optic tract produce 'homonymous hemianopia', specifically incongruous hemianopia.

Incongruity refers to asymmetry of visual field defects. Within the optic tract, the crossing nasal fibres and the uncrossed temporal fibres are separated anatomically. Thus visual field loss from lesions of the optic tract or the lateral geniculate body affect each eye differently, resulting in asymmetric field loss in each eye. Retrogeniculate homonymous field defects are almost always congruous, i.e. exactly similar because the nasal and temporal fibres from corresponding points of retina are closely associated.

Optic Radiations

Retinal fibres synapse at the lateral geniculate nucleus and project backwards as the 'geniculocalcarine radiations'. All the radiating fibres sweep laterally and inferiorly around the temporal horn of the lateral ventricle. The most anteroinferior fibres form the Meyer's loop, which contain projections of the inferior retinal fibres. Hence, lesions of the Meyer's loop, located primarily in the temporal lobe, produce 'congruous superior quadrantic visual field defect'.

More superiorly located parietal lobe lesions produce 'inferior homonymous quadrantic or hemianopic defects'.

Visual Cortex

The striate or primary visual cortex of humans occupies the medial and posterolateral part of the occipital lobe. Striate cortex is also found above, below and within the walls of the calcarine fissure. Topographically, central and paracentral zone of each hemifield is subserved by retinal axons that eventually terminate at the most posterior pole of the occipital lobe. A lesion here will produce 'homonymous central or paracentral hemianopic scotoma'. Such defects involve the central 5° to 10° of vision.

The other type of central defect, a 'homonymous hemianopia' with 'macular sparing' occurs with occipital lesions which spare the most posterior part of the occipital lobe.

The most peripheral portion of each hemifield which includes the temporal crescent, projects to the anterior lip of the calcarine fissure.

Lesions that spare the anterior cortex will cause homonymous hemianopias with 'sparing' of the temporal crescent. The temporal crescent is a 30° segment of monocular temporal field that begins 60° from fixation. It is entirely unshared and monocular, i.e. seen by one eye only.

These nasal retinal axons decussate in the optic chiasma and terminate in the most anterior part of the occipital cortex. Focal damage here would theoretically produce a monocular field defect that involved only the temporal crescent of the contralateral eye. Sparing of the temporal crescent, on the other hand, in the presence of congruous homonymous hemianopia, permits exact localization of the site lesion to the contralateral posterior occipital cortex.

Bilateral homonymous hemianopias result from bilateral, usually ischaemic lesions of the occipital cortex. If each homonymous defect involves the parafixation zone, the combined defects lead to a central scotoma and loss of central vision. Cortical blindness is characterized by:

1. Symmetrical loss of central field
2. Relatively 'normal' pupillary reactions
3. Denial of blindness
4. Bilateral occipital lesions in scans.

Accurate visual field testing and an intelligent interpretation of the results can provide extremely useful information regarding the site and type of lesion. As the human visual sensory pathways spans the brain from front to back, visual field anomalies are present in a wide variety of orbital and central nervous system disorders. Some common disorders in children include orbital and intracranial tumours, metastatic lesions, trauma, galactorrhoea syndromes, multiple sclerosis, malnutrition, hydrocephalus, drugs particularly ethambutol, and congenital vascular tumours (Fig. 15.2).

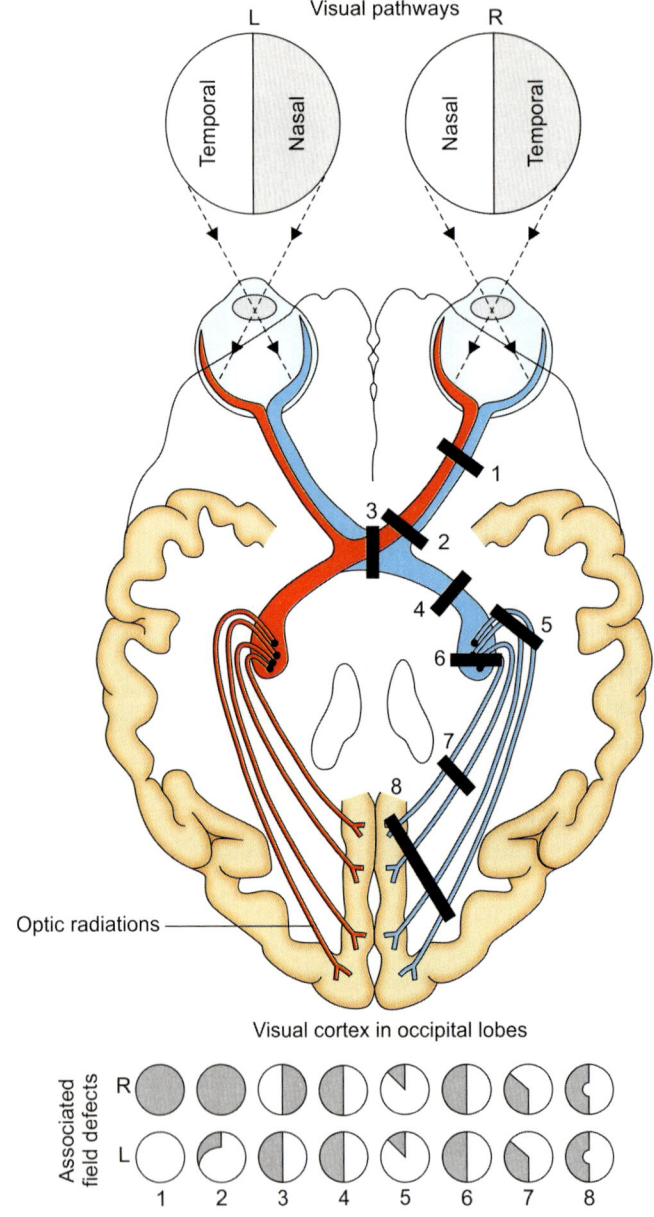

Fig. 15.2: Lesions at different places in the visual pathway to the visual cortex and associated field defects

TYPES OF PERIMETRY

It would be not out-of-place to give a brief account of types of perimetry used. There is a great variety in both the methods and apparatus used for assessing the field of vision. Basically, two methods of perimetry, i.e. kinetic and static, are used to detect the anomalies in the visual field.

Kinetic Perimetry

1. *Tangent screen:* The simplest form of perimetry is the tangent screen. It is a large black screen on which target (pins) attached to a black wand are moved from periphery to the centre of vision. These pins may be white or coloured.

2. *Goldman perimeter:* The Golmann perimetry is a manually operated device and consists of a white hollow spherical bowl positioned at a distance from the patient. The patient rests his chin on a chin-rest and fixes at the centre of the sphere, and an examiner moves a test light of variable size and intensity from the periphery to the centre. This manual perimetry has been largely replaced by automated perimetry.

3. *Automated perimetry:* Automated perimetry uses a mobile stimulus moved by the machine itself. The patient indicates when he sees the light by pressing a button. The use of white background and lights of incremental brightness is called 'white-on-white' perimetry. Though this is the most common type of method used, the brightness of target is affected by the white background and sensitivity becomes low and thus variability is relatively high. As many as 25–30% of photo-receptors may be lost this way before changes of visual field 'acuity' are detected. The patient sits in a small concave dome with chin on chin-rest and attention on a central target. The other eye is covered. A computer then shines light on the inside of the dome and the patient clicks the button whenever the light is seen.

4. *Semiautomated kinetic perimetry:* A semiautomated kinetic perimetry has been developed by Haag-Streit company and the equipment is termed as Octopus-900. It retains all the original characteristics of Goldmann manual perimeter.

Static Perimetry

Static perimetry tests different locations throughout the field one at a time. First, a dim light is projected at a particular location. If the person fails to detect, the light is made gradually brighter till it is seen. The minimum brightness required for detection is called the 'threshold' sensitivity level of that location. The procedure is repeated at several locations until the entire field is tested. Threshold detection is done generally by using static automated perimetry. It is useful for rapid perimetry and follow up of diseases involving deficits such as scotomas, loss of field, and eye diseases.

Numerous companies are in the market like Humphrey, Essilar, Oculus, Haag-Streit, etc. manufacturing static and kinetic perimeters.

Another type of field testing strategy is available called the 'frequency doubling technology' (FDT). This technique basically tests the ganglion cells sensitivity in the central field and is helpful in glaucoma.

Rehabilitation of the Visually Impaired Child

GENERAL CONSIDERATIONS

Visual impairment may take many forms and may be of varying degrees. Visual acuity alone is not always a good indicator or predictor of the degree of visual problems a person may have.

Somebody with relatively good visual acuity may have difficulty in doing fine work which his profession demands; or a person with 6/12 acuity may have extremely decreased peripheral vision and may be severely handicapped to go around.

Some people with moderate or severe visual impairment learn to use their residual vision, their remaining eyesight, to perform their daily tasks without relying on alternative methods.

The role of ophthalmologist is to maximize the functional level of the residual vision and make optimum use of this vision through different types of low vision aids. Other professionals can teach a visually handicapped person the use of non-optical means by which they can pursue the selected vocation and perform their daily routine.

For a visually impaired infant, recognition of parents voice will be noticed after 3 months of life; but a feel of parents face by sight is initiated very early in first month of life itself. As vision, which is a primary form of communication, is missing in a severely visually impaired infant or a small child, other forms of communication are also greatly delayed or impaired. As this child grows, social interactions are more complicated, as subtle visual clues are missing. Due to delays in child's communication development, they become disinterested in social activities and learning. These problems may be less severe, if the child is not totally blind and has some useful vision, which can be enhanced by suitable means. The purpose of this chapter is to highlight the problems of an visually impaired child, means to improve his remaining vision by optical devices and professional treatment as far as possible, understand the child's psychology, means to educate and provide vocational training to make him/her worthy and productive citizens in later life.

Children have a special place in rehabilitation programs. These are their formative years where not only education is important but also their psychological aspect has to be kept in mind. Children with worsening eyesight need special care and have to be prepared for a vocation they can pursue in later life to earn livelihood and integration in social circles.

Severe visual disability is a challenge for all health and associated professionals. Each child has to be assessed individually, taking into account the type and severity of visual impairment, the mental status, the family background, the type of education to be imparted, the type of optical aid required, and the type of vocational training needed for future employment.

There are nearly six million pre-school and school-age children who are blind or have low vision. 80% of these children live in developing countries, where less than 10% of these children have access to specialized education and training. Among the causes for this inequity are lack of early identification, referral and intervention; lack of trained personal and specialists; lack of appropriate equipment; lack of awareness in parents; limited government policy and implementation; and economic limitations of the affected families.

World Health Organization (WHO) uses the following classification for visual impairment (VI), after best correction:

1. Up to 6/24: Mild VI
2. Up to 6/60 : Moderate VI
3. 6/60 to 2/60: Severe VI
4. Less than 2/60: Near total VI

5. No PL–PR: Total blindness.
6. Visual fields in both eyes—less than 20°: Severe VI.
7. Visual fields less than 10° in both eyes: Near total VI.

These definitions were set by WHO in 1972, and since then there is ongoing discussions to reset the criteria. Whatever the criteria is decided upon, a person or a child who is unable to perform his daily routine with the best correction possible, comes into the category of severe visual impairment; and needs special care and rehabilitation.

Rehabilitation of a blind or visually handicapped child is a broad subject, and it will be easier to divide into relevant parts for better understanding.

The following sections would ease our process of understanding:

1. Psychosocial aspects of children, with low vision
2. Assessment of children with low vision
3. Treatment options
4. Training and rehabilitation services
5. Low vision aids
6. Assessment of children with multiple handicaps.

Psychosocial Problems

Children with worsening eyesight and prognosis of eventual blindness are at a high risk of succumbing to psychological distress. Data suggest that majority of children with congenital blindness die within two years of life. This is mostly due to neglect at home. Infections and other illnesses are other common causes, as medical attention of a blind child is last on the agenda of an impoverished family.

These observations advocate the establishment and extension of therapeutic programmes into preventive measures to avoid such catastrophes. Thus, there is need to incorporate other health professionals to cope with psychosocial aspects of a growing child as well as preparation for integration for future life.

At the same time, parents should be properly counselled about the ailment and its prognosis. Studies have demonstrated that rapid acceptance of the visual problem by parents and family has led to a better, more productive compliance of the rehabilitation programmes.

More importantly, a child should never be made to feel that the visual disability will make his/her life incapacitated and useless to the family and society. Time should be given to health and related professionals to understand the extent of disability, extra abilities the child has, and training avenues best suited to the child.

Another important aspect relates to the social environment, a visually handicapped child should never be isolated or debarred from mixing with other children. In social gatherings, the child should be allowed to mix and interact with people, encouraged to talk and discuss. Studies have shown that children with such handicaps, when allowed and encouraged to interact with other children and adults, have shown less mental stress and have learned to cope up with their problems.

As the child grows, he/she should be apprised of the visual problem, how to cope with that and accept the fact and seriously take the vocational training which the professionals advise. The patient should, at best, never be allowed to feel that his or her life is miserable and should be made to understand that with the suitable vocational training, they will lead a productive life independently.

As far as the future marital life is concerned—though this is not a subject to be incorporated here—but medical advice will not be out of place. In case marriage is contemplated, genetic assessment is essential, so that similar genetic disorder is not present in the prospective spouse.

Management of impending blindness or severely visually handicapped children is a challenge and is difficult. Lack of non-clinical training to provide severely visually impaired children with education and specialized vocational training to maintain safe, active and independent lifestyle, is unfortunately deficient in most countries and societies.

The unemployment rate in this group, despite special education, is 75 to 90%, and persons with low vision since childhood are five times more likely to be unemployed than general population. This high rate of unemployment in developing countries is the result of potential employers misconceptions; severe lack of proper vocational training and lack of technological resources.

Excluded from workplace and unable to be productive citizens, these people become discouraged and experience social and economical isolation and are prone to psychological disorders. These drawbacks deny millions of visually handicapped persons from engaging socially and be respected as productive members of society. If given proper education and tools to gain useful skill, the visually impaired children can realise their potential and contribute to the society, improving their future lives and bringing happiness for themselves and their families.

ASSESSMENT OF CHILDREN WITH LOW VISION

Generally speaking, the term low vision is referred for children when they are severely visually impaired even with conventional spectacles or contact lenses, but are able to use their vision for some daily activities.

Nevertheless, evaluation of a child with low vision or severe visual impairment is of paramount importance. After a correct diagnosis, efforts should be made to treat the disease as best as possible. Many a times, a multidisciplinary approach is needed. Parents should be explained fully and properly about the disorder and its possible modes of treatment. But simultaneously, they should also be apprised about the result of treatment and of prognosis.

The main causes of visual disability in children are nystagmus, congenital cataracts, albinism, cortical visual impairment (CVI), head injuries, high uncorrected refractive errors, and infective lesions involving the optic pathways. Some of these, when diagnosed early and treated effectively, have a reasonably good prognosis; but severe albinism and CVI pose a major challenge. Treatment options are limited in these conditions and by the time a child is old enough to initiate treatment, deep irreversible amblyopia has already set in.

In the above mentioned conditions, sincere assessment of the residual visual acuity with the age matched testing devices, is utmost necessity.

Also a child's other capabilities and talents should be assessed. Suitable visual aids, for both near and distance should be tried to improve his/her residual vision, and then a vocational training, best suited for, should be initiated.

If the child's intelligence is high or inclination towards learning is appreciable, then further education avenues should be provided with special learning devices.

TREATMENT OPTIONS

A brief overview of treatment options would not be out-of-place for mentioning.

1. *Congenital cataracts* still pose a major cause of severe visual impairment.

   As a rule of thumb, uniocular or binocular congenital cataracts, obscuring the vision, should be promptly treated. There are ample studies which advocate removing of the cataract by three months of life. IOL implantation, at what age, of what type and power, is highly controversial. But removal of dense cataract, as early as possible, is universally accepted. Management of an aphakic infant or child is the next challenge. It requires long, painstaking and sincere efforts from both an ophthalmologist and parents perspective. It also requires highly trained and motivated paediatric ophthalmologist to venture on this management.

2. *Congenital nystagmus* is another area, where no ophthalmologist dares to dwell. The reasons and causes of nystagmus are not required here, but every paediatric ophthalmologist must be aware of the type of nystagmus the child has, and the best optical, conventional or surgical treatment required for the condition which may improve vision.

3. *High uncorrected refractive errors* is not only a major cause of deep amblyopia, both unilateral or bilateral, but also strabismus, nystagmus, and psychological disorders. It is a misfortune that even fully educated ophthalmologists, either

do not know or take casually, to do a proper refraction of a small child. Prescription of spectacles in various types of refractive errors requires deep thought and experience. It is of concern that a child devoid of a proper spectacle continues to reel under headaches and other symptoms of ocular asthenopia and also blurred visual acuity.

It is stressed here that children not only should be properly refracted, but their spectacles should be appropriately ordered according to the type of refractive error; and assessed frequently in cases of rapid change in their refractive errors.

4. *Cortical visual impairment (CVI)* is a serious problem. Most of these cases are of neonatal birth asphyxias, birth trauma, or perinatal infections. Whatever the cause may be, a very careful ophthalmic examination is mandatory to rule out any ocular morbidity. Once this is ascertained, a paediatric neurological examination including brain scans are important to fix the diagnosis. Once the diagnosis is finalized, time should be given for as much spontaneous recovery as possible; and then management on lines of severe low vision should be initiated.

5. The other important reason for impaired vision in infants and children are perinatal or childhood cerebral infections like viral encephalitis or microbial meningitis. A common unfortunate state here is that a paediatrician is totally engrossed in managing the disease, oblivious (probably unknowingly), that a simultaneous injury is also occurring to the visual pathways. And by the time, damage to vision is noted, the damage is irreversible.

These are the areas where a conscious effort should be made by combined multidisciplinary effort to save life and also save sight!

6. *Albinism* is another disorder seriously affecting vision which demands a passing note. The term albinism comes from the Latin word *'albus'* meaning 'white', and in year 1908 was first scientifically described by Garrod.

It is essentially a group of hereditary disorders involving the synthesis and distribution of melanin. Clinically, albinism presents as a pigmentation abnormality of skin, hair, and/or eyes. These are broadly of two types: (1) Oculocutaneous albinism, and (2) ocular albinism, involving the eyes only. In both categories, the primary morbidity is eye related. Ocular signs and symptoms include severe photophobia, refractive errors, nystagmus, strabismus, foveal hypoplasia, and abnormal decussation of optic nerve fibres. These ocular manifestations are almost always present in both types of albinism.

The reason for this elaboration is that an ophthalmologist should be aware that after all his efforts to correct refractive error, nystagmus or photophobia (by prescribing dark lenses), some amount of visual defect still remains, due to the anatomical disorder, he need not be discouraged.

TRAINING AND REHABILITATION SERVICES

The education programmes should include development of skills which will help the visually handicapped. These skills may include reading and writing in Braille, travel skills—known as 'orientation and mobility' techniques (O and M); and optimum use of the low vision.

Some children may attend special schools which have special programmes for the visually impaired. Here programmes are tailored towards students with single or multiple disabilities, which also include life-long functional programmes.

A child has to be individually assessed and any inherent talent or skill should be unearthed. Such children may be groomed in their skill and encouraged for vocational development in that field for their livelihood. For example, a student with intelligence may be inclined to pursue further education and may need books transcribed into Braille or a student with low vision may need a 'low vision device' such as a magnifier or a CCTV to complete the studies.

In essence, individual child has to be carefully and thoroughly examined by a team comprising of an ophthalmologist, social worker, psychologist and a person trained to impart special education. This team assesses the gravity of visual impairment; the students' abilities, strengths and needs; determines the most appropriate educational placements; sets educational goals and objectives; and specifies the special educational and related services for the child.

At the same time, some recreational facilities should also be provided to these children. As already stated earlier, a child should not feel isolated and neglected, thus some recreational facilities, suitable for the type of disability, should be made available in schools.

The plan should be to provide integrated education along with specialized training to aid in the development of critical life skills for adulthood.

The following needs should be addressed:

1. *Awareness:* Families, healthcare professionals, and educators are simply not aware that visually handicapped children can successfully complete their education.

2. *Education:* The majority of children with mild to moderate low vision can be assimilated in a normal school, if teachers are imparted some extra training to cater to the needs of visually handicapped. Special schools for severely handicapped children should have all the gadgets and tools for education like Braille books, CCTV monitors, low vision aids, etc.

3. *Trained teachers:* Caring and teaching of visually handicapped children requires teachers with special training. Unfortunately, such training centres are lacking and thus there is scarcity of such teachers.

Rehabilitation

Rehabilitation consists of a wide range of clinical therapy and non-clinical training to provide for children who are blind or have very low vision.

Though rehabilitation cannot restore the lost sight, but it can help maximize any remaining vision so that these children can learn, travel safely, take care of their needs, meet their educational goals, and become independent citizens in later life.

Blindness does not have to be a barrier to successful employment. The services for visually handicapped should include counselling and guidance; mental restoration (psychological confidence building); training and providing means for higher education; job development and job placement; and follow-up services to ensure that the rehabilitated person is performing satisfactorily in the job. There are a variety of jobs suited for a visually impaired, e.g. stenotypist, teacher, musician, councillor, receptionist, computer programmer, etc.

Professional Development

This is probably the most critical area of their lives.

Children who are blind or severely visually handicapped need to learn as best as they can with whatever tools available to increase their work readiness. Students can involve in 'oral education', or e-learning and virtual job coaching.

Special Braille keyboards with computer screens are now available where partially sighted children can type in Braille and visualize letters on screen with 'enlarged fonts' and also hear and speak what they are typing. Once they learn typing, these children can take jobs in offices where typing computers are made available in Braille.

For children who have special skills of music or singing can learn these in music classes and take this vocation as their livelihood. There are number of examples of such people in the world.

Vocational training or artisan training in different walks of life can be taught to earn a permanent livelihood (Fig. 16.1).

Learning

Children with low vision have reading delays and are slow at learning. It is to be remembered that over 70% of learning is through sight, and most of the basic learning is maximum in first 7 years of life. A child with low vision is at a loss to read and write by sight. Studies have shown that in such cases, 'phonic' bases learning has been very fruitful. Engaging in phonic instructions is multisensory, highly motivating, and helps in rapid learning.

Typically, children are first taught the most frequent sounds, i.e. short vowel sounds, then taught to blend sounds of three letter words like cat, dog, etc. Then very enlarged print is shown to

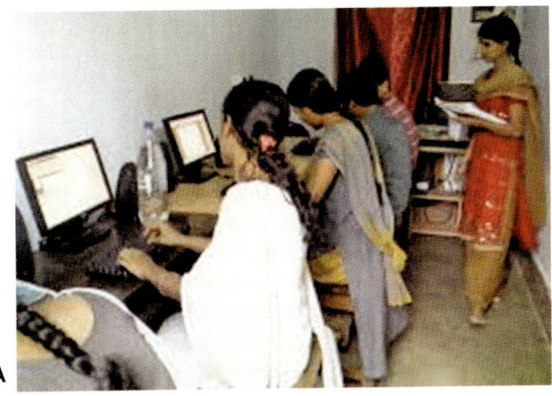

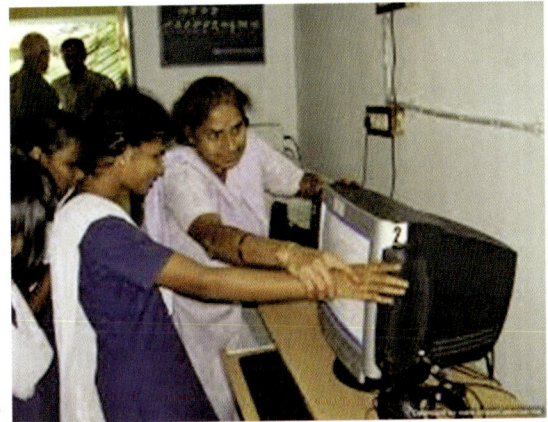

Fig. 16.1A and B: Training classes with computers in Braille script

understand what they have learned phonically. This 'kinesthical' technique is very useful to compliment phonically learned words. Gradually, this kinesthical learning is incorporated in sentences. It is also important that the written material is not in capital letters, as routine sentences are not in capital letters! The most relevant and useful written material is the Braille script.

The Braille Script

This system was invented and instituted by Louise Braille, who became totally blind at the age of 12 years! But who taught the world that a blind person can also read and write and lead a productive life.

The Braille script constitutes of 'raised knobs' on a sheet; the knobs have a characteristic configuration and by recognising the configuration of each knob, a low vision child can read letters. There are type-writters and now computer with Braille fonts.

Books are available with Braille pattern pictures and fonts to read stories and understand pictures. These are on 'tactile' pattern (Fig. 16.2).

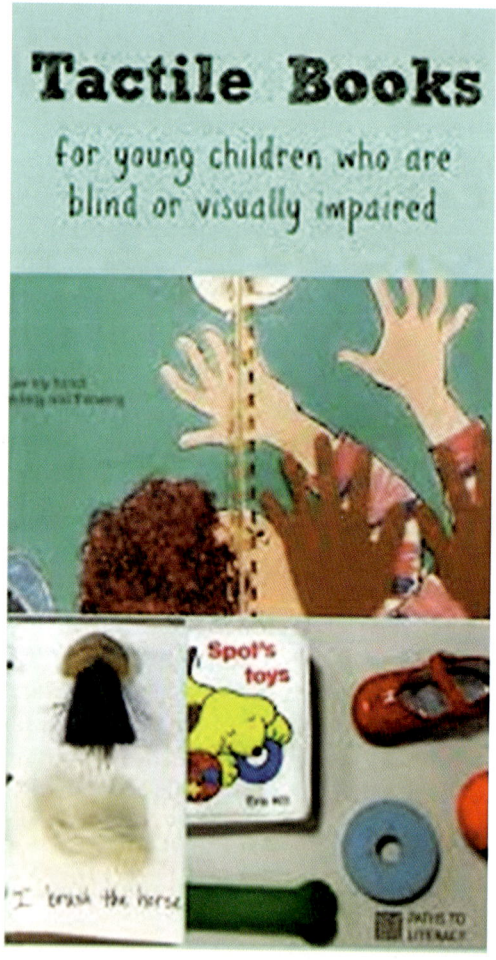

Fig. 16.2: Tactile Books in Braille script for learnaing

Mobility

The following narration is common for children as well as adults, and is taken together because what children learn at their age, is followed and refined throughout life.

Many people with severe low vision can travel independently using a wide range of devices and technique. Orientation and mobility are learned by training from specialists, to move around confidently at home and in community.

Tools such as 'white cane with a red tip'— an international symbol of blindness—may be used to facilitate mobility. A number of people employ 'guide dogs' to help them negotiate obstacles. Some blind persons develop skills in 'echo-locating', which employees special sound produced by mouth and listening to the returning echoes. It has been shown that echolocation experts use what is normally the 'visual' part of the brain to process the echoes.

All above mechanisms are areas where a blind person is trained right from childhood.

Magnification Devices

Most visually handicapped children who are not totally blind, can read print of normal size by enlarging them by 'magnification'. A variety of magnification devices are available, some hand-held and some desk mounted.

Distance viewing: Telescopic devices are available which enables a person to bring the distant object near, thus enabling them to see. Uniocular as well as binocular telescopes are available. The only disadvantage is that the field of vision becomes very restricted.

Similarly for reading, hand-held 'magnifiers' can be used to enlarge the reading material and making it readable. Children with multiple deficits, where hand coordination is lacking, 'fixed-distance' desk mounted magnifiers can be used for learning. One of the simplest way to enhance magnification is to provide spectacles with 'high plus lenses', which sufficiently magnifies the script for partially visual impaired children (Fig. 16.3).

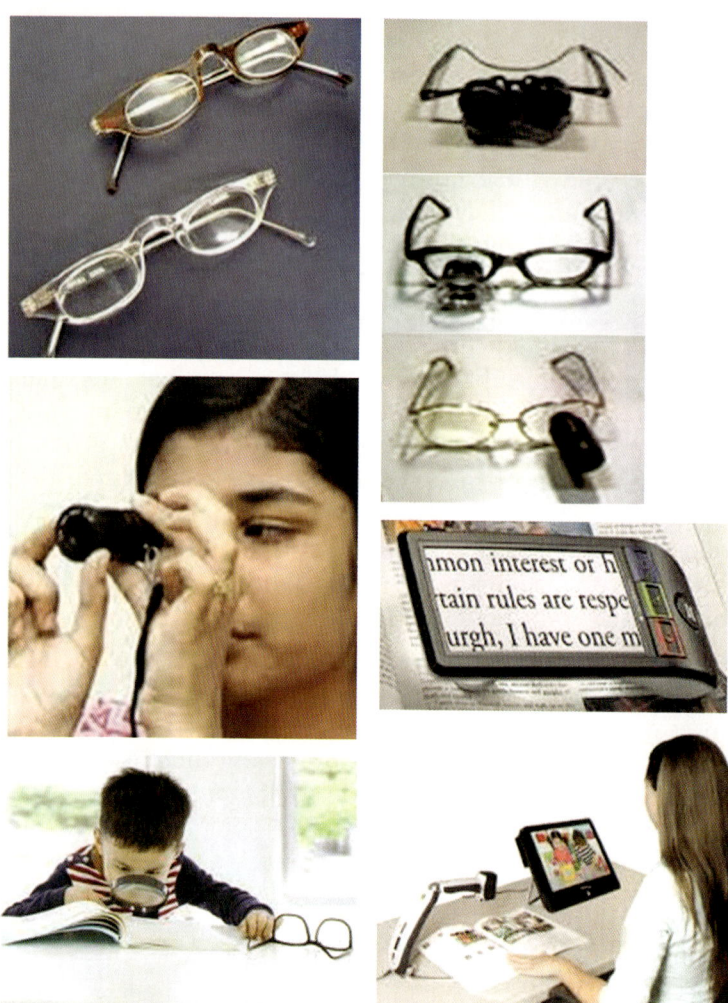

Fig. 16.3: Various types of low-vision devices.

Today, computers are available where reading 'font' can be sufficiently enlarged, for a child or an adult, to read and learn.

In short, the following devices are commercially available optical devices:

1. Monocular telescopes

2. Spectacle-mounted telescope
3. Bioptic telescopes.

These telescopes differ than the conventional ones as they allow the user to walk and travel, without much reduction of visual fields.

Near devices: Magnifiers:
- Hand-held
- Stand magnifiers—fixed distance
- Illuminated magnifiers
- CCTV systems—having enlarged font facility.
- Speech integrated CCTV systems.

Other aids:
- Some bank notes in some countries have 'engraved areas', especially the denomination, where the amount can be recognised by touch.
- Some coins too have such type of arrangement.
- Wrist watches, table clocks, table calenders, and similar host of domestic items can be specially engraved to be recognised by touch.

Development of Special Senses

Touch: Touch is an important aspect of how a visually handicapped child uses to identify his surroundings. Touch gives information about the shape, size, texture, temperature, and many other information.

Children, from very early age, develop this very important aspect of knowledge.

Smell: Smell can be used, as is used by normal persons, to identify areas or recall of a particular place.

Children with multiple disabilities: Children with multiple disabilities should be enrolled in special schools with specialized equipment, and personnel with special training. A medical specialist should be available for regular supervision from time-to-time.

Unfortunately, these types of specialized institutions are lacking in India.

Different disabilities are treated at different institutions, without any coordination and lacking in integrated management of a visually handicapped child with other disabilities.

Nevertheless, vision—which is of paramount importance for learning and development of a child—should be managed on priority basis by a team of experts.

A Blind Child:
Role of the Clinician

There are numerous examples of disharmony between parents of a blind child and the clinician. Declaring that the infant or child is blind and there is no treatment, is one of the most disturbing moments in a physician's career.

The impact of blindness upon all family members is tremendous. One of the most treasured moments in a parents' life is the birth of a healthy baby. The first smile of a newborn is the most treasured moment for a parent. Parents start loving their baby long before it is born. Their baby is all their dreams, fantasies, and expectations. It is their future and their hope.

Imagine when they hear that their baby is 'born blind'. It has the most devastating effect and their lives are shattered. They see an unknown, unseen enemy in front of them whom they cannot fight. They are brimmed with anger and revenge but oblivious against whom to vent their rage.

A parent experiences one of life's most devastating losses when they learn that their child cannot see. Such a loss shatters the dreams which are most basic to human nature. Such a loss as blindness for an expected perfect baby is a mental trauma unsurpassed for the family.

The kinds of feeling parents have in response to their child's disability may be confusing to them. Denial is the first response. They will not believe their ears and understandably question number of times. They may seek multiple opinions. In the end, they feel helpless, fear, sadness, guilt, and disappointment. They are in shock and feel lost as there is nothing they can do.

Another important and universal reaction the parents have, sooner or later, is an overwhelming need to know what went wrong! And to know the reason of the catastrophe.

So many things come to the mind of the mother, for example, heavy work during pregnancy, fever, any illness, tobacco or alcohol intake, the list is endless. Some of the reasons can be explainable from medical point of view, while many have no obvious explanation. To some, religious belief gives comfort, while some feel solace in destiny. But to most, it is a nightmare which keeps on coming every night for rest of their lives.

BREAKING THE NEWS

Clinicians are often unaware that their role has a direct impact on the adaptation process for the family. The way the doctor presents the diagnosis to the parents is crucial. For long many years, the family will remember not just what they were told but how it was conveyed to them. The interaction between doctor and parents in such circumstances is very important and should be based on consideration, truth, clarity, compassion, awareness, and professional kindness.

Truth: It is understandably difficult for the doctor to give a bad news to the patient. But eventually it will have to be spelt out. One can start gently by saying that "your child has a serious disease. He is not able to see. But we will try and find some solution."

This will not create a sudden impact. This envisages many messages. Firstly, you have not uttered the word 'blind'—which has tremendous implications. Secondly, you have said there could be some solution later on (which implies special education in a blind school and vocational training); and also you have not uttered the name of blind-school. As one great physician said, "There are many ways to say the same thing. Truth does not mean brutality."

Clarity: Give information in a plain language. Parents are already anxious and will not apprehend medical jargon.

Too much explanation is not needed as the doctor may inadvertently spell out some unwanted words. If required, the parents can be called at some other time, if they need more explanation.

Awareness: Keep an eye on how the family is reacting. Understand that you are giving a diagnosis of which there is no cure. If your diagnosis has suddenly alarmed the parents, stop at this moment. Let them overcome the initial impact and offer them water or coffee, and come back after some time later to complete your statement.

Compassion: Always in such situations, compassion is the greatest virtue. Express sorry and sadness, and feel concerned about the ailment as if this has happened to your very close kin.

Taking the hand of parent in your hand and expressing grief, goes a long way in comforting the parents. This is a bad moment in your professional career but you yourself should be calm and composed. There could be a chance where the parent may blame the perinatal events for the catastrophe and may point finger at the obstetrician. Do not, at any point, reverberate the same feeling as the parent. On the contrary, bypass if any such event has occurred because you do not know the real-time events at that time.

Trust: Parents should trust you in not only what you are saying but for any help they may require in future. They must trust you that you are honest with them at all times.

Accessibility: Parents may not absorb the impact at once. As already said, they may come back to you for further counselling. May be they have not understood the diagnosis at that stressful moment and come back later. They may also seek further advice. In all these situations, you must be available to give professional help as much as possible. Be co-operative and do not express that your work is done and you are no more concerned with the patient.

Professional kindness: Above all, professional kindness is of paramount importance. It is that single virtue of highest order and encompasses all what is discussed above. It is a tool, a means of dealing with patients in a kind and humane way. Professional kindness helps parents to understand their child's ailment and to cope with it. They acknowledge that you care and are concerned about the child's welfare. Good advice for their future regarding education and vocation will go a long way in comforting them.

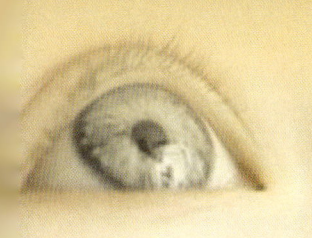

Index

293